Medical English

R. Ribes · P. R. Ros

Ramón Ribes · Pablo R. Ros

Medical English

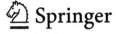 Springer

Ramón Ribes, MD, PhD
Hospital Reina Sofia
Servicio de Radiología
Avda. Menéndez Pidal s/n.
Córdoba 14005, Spain

Pablo R. Ros, MD, MPH
Professor of Radiology, Harvard Medical School
Executive Vice Chairman and Associate Radiologist-in-Chief,
Brigham and Women's Hospital
Chief, Division of Radiology, Dana-Farber Cancer Institute
Harvard Medical School
75 Francis St.
Boston, MA 02115, USA

ISBN-10   3-540-25428-5 Springer Berlin Heidelberg New York
ISBN-13   978-3-540-25428-7 Springer Berlin Heidelberg New York

Library of Congress Control Number: 2005928947

Springer is a part of Springer Science+Business Media

springeronline.com

© Springer-Verlag Berlin · Heidelberg 2006
Printed in Germany

Editor: Dr. Ute Heilmann, Springer-Verlag
Desk Editor: Wilma McHugh, Springer-Verlag
Production: Pro Edit GmbH, Elke Beul-Göhringer, Heidelberg, Germany
Typesetting: K+V Fotosatz GmbH, Beerfelden
Cover design: Estudio Calamar, F. Steinen-Broo, Pau/Girona, Spain

24/3151/beu-göh – 5 4 3 2 1 0 – Printed on acid-free paper

To my father, Ramón Ribes Blanquer,
for teaching me to seize every moment of life.

R. Ribes

To Silvia...
My guide, my love, my life.

P. R. Ros

Foreword

It has been a long time since English became the language of science. Today, in modern medical practice, and here I include all specialties, medical professionals are constantly exposed, either when searching the literature or attending meetings, to the English language. The scientific importance of English is such that, whenever I have a meeting with my residents – and I have many, both residents and meetings – I find myself emphasizing, over and over again, the need for them to learn English. I may be exaggerating, but I do think that unless you know enough English to read the medical literature, it is almost impossible to keep up to date with medical advances. I honestly feel that English should be a compulsory subject at medical school.

Whenever I attend international medical meetings, and see how some colleagues struggle, not only in trying to converse with their English-speaking counterparts but also in trying to understand their lectures, I strongly feel that we should try to do something to prevent this from happening in future generations.

Many of us who completed our medical training in English-speaking countries still remember how much we suffered during our first weeks on call. Local idioms and colloquialisms on the one hand, and medical abbreviations on the other, drove us to the brink of despair. This work is like a breath of fresh air with regard to the idiomatic problem affecting so many of our young, and not so young, doctors. This book will not only help them to improve their English but will also introduce them to the world of medical jargon. I wish I had had such a book when, as a young resident, I had to present a case, or even later on, when I was first asked to chair a session at an international English-speaking meeting! This volume would have been a godsend in both situations, and in many others. I am confident that in the near future many health care professionals will benefit from the book. Here I mean not only those who work in the English-speaking world but also those practicing in their own countries.

I sincerely congratulate the authors on writing such a necessary book, which will certainly improve the linguistic training of many doctors. It was a pleasure for me to review the manuscript and it has been a great honor to write this foreword. I wish I could have written such a book myself.

Dr. Javier Lucaya
Chairman of Radiology, Vall d'Hebrón Hospital, Barcelona, Spain, July 2005

Preface

The need for English as a professional language in medicine is nowadays beyond doubt. Scientific literature and the internet are just two examples that reveal the overriding necessity for understanding and expressing ourselves in written and spoken English.

The formal teaching of English, overloaded to excess with theoretical content, does not enable us to keep in touch, using English as a common language, with other professionals abroad, and thus development opportunities are continually wasted. With this manual, we intend to help overcome this state of affairs.

Most interns and staff members withdrew from the formal learning of English a long time ago, and English has become an everlasting failed subject. Only the most determined have continued studying, with more tenacity than method, but unfortunately, in most cases with little if any success. Many colleagues have thrown in the towel. Many have desisted from attending, if indeed they ever tried to attend, international courses and congresses, and among the reduced group of those who dare, participation is very limited on most occasions.

It is true that both components of language, sensory and motor, have to be integrated into our brain from childhood, if not, then the older we get, the less natural language learning becomes. It is no less true that the conviction that the use of English will bring extraordinary advantages may become a strong extra motivation. The US President William J. Clinton said, on a certain occasion, that in the future, mankind could be divided into "educated and non-educated people", and that the imaginary boundary that would separate the two worlds would be knowledge of English and computers.

No-one would pretend that non-English-speaking physicians could be, in the use of their mother tongue, up to their North American and British colleagues. But that is no obstacle to achieving a level comparable to that of other colleagues coming from countries other than English-speaking countries.

With this manual, we intend to turn what until now has been considered a wearisome task into an amusing close-up inside professional medical English, but also bearing in mind that no result is achieved without effort. The classic manual entitled "English without effort" should, in our opinion, be changed to "English without sacrifice".

We recommend a thorough study of the unit "Grammar in Use", which was created using medical terminology, because without such practical grammar notions, we cannot build up our knowledge of English. Our aim should not be just to make ourselves understood, but to do so at the appropriate levels of fluency and correctness.

It is obvious that using English outside English-speaking countries entails an additional effort in keeping ourselves up to date. The international press, movies (original versions are recommended or, for intermediate levels, subtitles in English) and cable television are useful allies. Without them, English will keep on being that reviled failed subject. Following international news through British and American news bulletins allows us to optimize our time and welcome English into our tight schedule as well as to receive useful information.

For many years, I have kept in touch with written and spoken English, although at a distance, through buying an American or British newspaper once a week, daily cable TV news reports and original version movies at the weekends. But without any doubt, the greatest stimulus came through my six month rotation at the Brigham and Women's Hospital (Harvard Medical School) at Boston, Massachusetts, as a research fellow.

Only through assisting at international meetings, courses and lectures, can the use of English as a professional language be perceived as a pressing need, thus making possible maintenance of the motivation required for this hard task.

As in many other subjects, the study that initially demands a high level of discipline may, as the learning goes on, become something agreeable, and the need to study may, for those who are enthusiastic, turn into devotion.

Ramón Ribes, MD, PhD
July 2005

Preface

As a non-native English speaker, practicing medicine in the United States for many years, I am delighted *Medical English* is seeing the light. I can vividly remember the fear I had when at the beginning of my residency I had to dictate complex radiology reports *in English*! I realized the importance of language accuracy so that the appropriate imaging findings were described in the report and the final diagnosis was correctly stated. Appropriate wording obviously needed to convey the message to the referring clinicians so patients could have adequate management.

The next step was to conquer public speaking *in English*! This started with presenting interesting cases in small groups, later in interdisciplinary conferences, and eventually lecturing to other colleagues and trainees with audiences of variable size.

Since I chose an academic career, I have had the opportunity to train many physicians and many of them have been, like me, non-native English speakers. Maybe because we have had this point in common it has been easier for me to try to help in the way they communicate in English.

I like to teach proper English construction and pronunciation to our non-native English speaking trainees. Since in medicine there are many terms written similarly but pronounced differently in languages other than English, it is easy to get confused. As was done for me when I was a resident, I like to write on a piece of paper words that our trainees mispronounce or sentences that are not in proper English. Then I ask the non-native English speaking physician to read out loud the word or the sentence and make corrections. By the same token I am pleased when a native English speaker is kind enough to tell me words I still mispronounce or sentences I misconstruct.

Therefore, when Dr. Ramon Ribes was a research fellow working with me a few years ago and discussed the idea of putting together this manual, I was engaged by it and gave my full support.

Now, Medical English is a reality and we hope our readers will find it both useful and fun. The idea is to condense in an easy to read volume the knowledge and the experience accumulated trying to practice medicine in English. Enjoy it!

Pablo R. Ros, MD, MPH
July 2005

Contents

Unit I
Reading, Listening, Talking and Writing. Self-evaluation

Unit II
Grammar in Use

Unit III
Scientific Literature

Unit IV
Talks and Courses

Unit V
Some of the Most Frequent Mistakes
Made by Doctors Speaking in English

Unit VI
Latin and Greek Terminology

Unit VII
Acronyms and Abbreviations

Unit VIII
The Clinical History

Unit IX
Conversation Survival Guide

Contributors

JOSÉ MARÍA MARTOS
Radiology resident
at Reina Sofía Hospital
Córdoba, Spain
contributed to the preparation
of Units 2, 6, 7, 8, and 9.

JOSÉ LUIS SANCHO
Radiologist at Alto Guadalquivir
Hospital
Andújar (Jaén), Spain
contributed to the preparation
of Units 2, 6, 7, and 8.

CONCHA ORTÍZ
Philologist and interpreter
contributed to the preparation
of Units 4, 5, and 7.

ELOISA FELIÚ
Radiologist at the INSCANNER
MR Unit, Alicante, Spain
contributed to the preparation
of Unit 3.

SANTIAGO TOFÉ
Endocrinologist at Son Dureta
Hospital
Palma de Mallorca, Spain
contributed to the preparation
of Units 2 and 3.

JOSÉ MARÍA VIDA
Radiologist at Montilla Hospital
Córdoba, Spain
contributed to the preparation
of Units 6 and 7.

PEDRO ARANDA
Cardiovascular surgery resident
at Reina Sofía Hospital
Córdoba, Spain
contributed to the preparation
of Unit 9.

ANTONIO LUNA
Radiologist at SERCOSA
Jaén, Spain
contributed to the preparation
of Unit 6.

FRANCISCO TRIVIÑO
Radiology resident
at Reina Sofía Hospital
Córdoba, Spain
contributed to the preparation
of Unit 9.

ROCÍO DÍAZ
Radiology resident
at Reina Sofía Hospital
Córdoba, Spain
contributed to the preparation
of Unit 2.

FRANCISCO MUÑOZ
Family doctor and ENT consultant
at Reina Sofía Hospital
Córdoba, Spain
drew the cartoons.

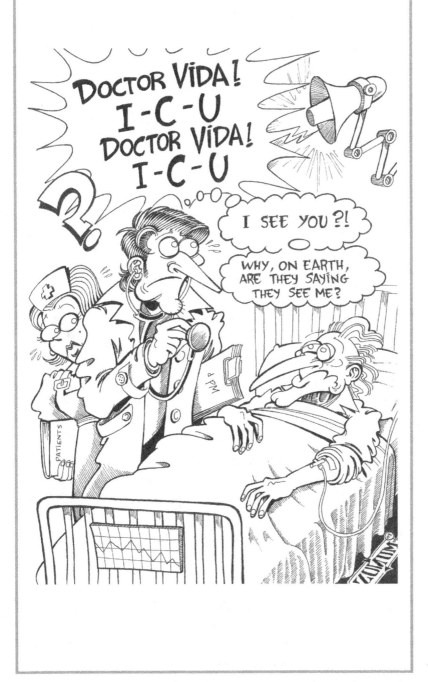

Unit I   Reading, Listening, Talking and Writing. Self-evaluation

Introduction

This is an introductory chapter that presents a new point of view about the learning of professional English. Knowledge of medical English has been one of the historical disadvantages of health-care professionals from non-English-speaking countries, and this manual focuses on a practical approach to the English that health-care professionals in general, and physicians in particular, need.

Reading has to be considered the first step in the learning of a foreign language. Reading professional manuscripts is an essential task for everyone who wants to be informed, and medicine is a constantly changing environment where, unfortunately, being uninformed is extraordinarily simple.

Familiarity with some terms and grammatical structures will make articles easier to read and, therefore, allow you to get more accurate information. The goal in terms of reading would be to feel as comfortable with English papers as you are with those written in your native tongue.

In the beginning, reading out loud will be a troublesome task because there are a lot of words that, knowing their meaning and even their spelling, are very difficult to pronounce. As in many other aspects of life, two paths can be taken; the easy one is to avoid this demanding exercise and the difficult, and more profitable one, requires using the dictionary to look up not only the unknown words for their meaning but also the known ones for their pronunciation.

Bear in mind that the lack of pronunciation skill is one of the greatest enemies of self-confidence when speaking a foreign language. If the lectures we attend were subtitled, most of us would understand them because our ability to understand what we read is much greater than our ability to speak and understand what we listen to.

Being aware of this fact can represent a vital step in your training; reading out loud will triple a reading exercise that suddenly will become a reading–listening–speaking one. When I began this kind of exercise I was barely able to read a few lines without consulting the dictionary; it was terribly hard and to read a few paragraphs took several hours. Do not give up, time and patience will provide amazing results.

Take into account that the terminology is not so extensive in your specialty although it can seem unbearable at the beginning. As you continue with this exercise, words you cannot pronounce will decrease and you will be able to read medical papers in a straightforward manner. Remember to begin with that the only words that you will have to practice are those that belong to your specialty and are going to be used on a routine basis, and the colloquial words that we have included in our conversation guide (Unit IX).

Listening is, probably, the most important skill to optimize. When we attend a conference, most of us will not ask any questions. Without talking you can get valuable information in a congress if you understand what speakers are saying. Even in our own language our capacity to understand is greater than our ability to talk. We can understand almost everything in a complex talk about an unknown subject about which we would be barely able to say a few sentences.

To develop listening skills is, therefore, paramount in our careers. The first step could be listening to ourselves reading out loud. There are some other exercises to be done. Watching movies with English subtitles is another essential activity. Unless you have got an outstanding English level, movies without subtitles will be discouraging. I encourage you to watch TV news bulletins; although they are obviously not subtitled they tend to be easier to understand.

Speaking in English must be the next step. Once you can read and understand what others say, you will feel the pressing need to say what you think. But this need will only appear if you have developed the ability to speak in a correct manner, otherwise you will avoid it for fear of being considered not fluent in English.

To be fluent in a foreign language is an extremely demanding task, and when we attend an international congress our lack of confidence in English prevents us from communicating with colleagues from other countries. As professionals we cannot speak poorly such that we can only just be understood; on the contrary, we need to express our opinions and feelings in a correct and consistent manner. If you have attended international courses you will agree that many non-English-speaking doctors try to stay together, becoming an island within an ocean of communications and relationships between professionals (doctors, nurses, technicians, salesmen, etc). Incredibly, many health-care professionals come back from international congresses not only without having given a talk but without having spoken English at all.

I will give you a piece of advice. When you arrive at a meeting begin talking to colleagues from non-English-speaking countries. It is easier to understand them and you will notice that they have the same difficulty as you do. They also make mistakes and their level may not be much higher than yours. You will feel comfortable talking to them and your mistakes (everybody makes mistakes even speaking in their own language) will not prevent you from keeping on talking. This will allow you to break the vicious circle that has kept you professionally deaf and dumb at international meetings.

Talking to doctors, nurses, technicians, and others, in the hospital is in the beginning a troublesome task. This is probably one of the most challenging topics for health-care professionals in foreign hospitals because, to be honest, there is only one way to become familiar with the hospital jargon, with the terminology used by doctors, nurses, technicians, and patients, and that is to work at an American or British hospital.

There are many words you realize you do not know during your first days rotating in a foreign hospital – words as simple as "stretcher", "coat", "white jacket", "white coat" or "ward" can be absolutely new for you in English – and expressions such as "to be paged" or "to be on-call" can be impossible to understand at the beginning. These words and sentences are "so inside" the hospital, so deep in the core of hospital terminology, that neither medical books nor medical dictionaries include them among their "more academic" terms.

Although we positively know that our approach to medical terminology is going to be just an introduction, just a preliminary approach to hospital terminology, we also know that the first step is the most important one and the one where more help is needed. Indeed, this whole manual is an introduction and you will have to write your own personal medical English book because medicine is so specialized nowadays that even physicians of the same specialty have difficulty in understanding each others talking about specific matters. (I myself am much more fluent in MR and interventional radiology than in ultrasound or CT.) That happens in English as well as in your mother tongue; we can only be really fluent in what we are speaking about everyday.

Those of you who have been in an American or British hospital know how important it is to get a white coat as soon as possible. Without a white coat nobody will identify you as a doctor and the chances are that "for security reasons" someone may invite you to leave the medical center. But ... who dares to ask for a coat without knowing how to say it in English? and, what is worse, without wanting anybody else to realize that you do not know this particular word. Will anybody trust me if they realize that I do not know words as simple as coat? Will anybody give me the opportunity of co-writing an article with such a level of English? What are they going to think of me? All these questions get into your mind without knowing at that time that probably nobody is going to waste a second thinking of you, your English level or any other stupid thought of yours. Anyway, the first two things to get once you are in an American hospital are an identification card and a white coat (remember that in American hospitals there are two kinds of coats, namely short coats and long coats, and the term "butcher-length coat" is likely to appear in your life).

The first days of rotation are generally a complete mess; there are so many things in your mind that "medicine", that is supposed to be the reason why you are so far from home, is pretty much at the bottom of your priorities.

If you are planning to do a rotation abroad and want to accept a piece of advice, take your time to get your "collateral affairs" in order and arrive in the city a week earlier to arrange "those little things" that make us look so foolish at the beginning. On my first day of rotation at the Brigham and Women's Hospital I did not know where I was going to sleep that night. Can you imagine in such a situation my level of concentration on the differences between adrenal adenomas and metastases on "in-" and "out-of-phase" MR sequences? So, do not make the same mistake, and get rid of "those little things" before the beginning of your rotation. Do not forget that the first impression could be the only one left and during your very first few days you may be creating in others that definitive "first impression".

The lack of a basic vocabulary made up of usual words and sentences will undermine your ability to optimize your time at the hospital, so do not miss the opportunity of being as fluent as possible in a competitive environment where time counts so much.

What do physicians talk about? Docs talk about patients, calls, residents if they are attendings, and attendings if they are residents, attendings from either their or other departments, colleagues of the same specialty, talks, courses, papers...

Sometimes you know the basic word or words and the key concept and you would be able to understand a sentence including them but you do not know the phrasal verbs and the usual expressions in which these known terms are embedded, so you could not make natural sentences with them. Remember once more that the goal is not just to be understood but to express your thoughts and feelings in a proper manner, at the appropriate level of English expected of a well-trained physician.

To know the word "blood" will allow you in a certain context to understand the sentence "the residents are *drawing blood* early in the morning", but ... would you have been able to say it? Probably not. To be "on-call" or "off-call" are usual expressions that you probably have not heard of before because in papers nobody talks about calls.

Try to imagine yourself taking part in these conversations. Write your own sentences and repeat them up to the point in which they become automatic. At the beginning do it with simple short questions such as "do you know what I mean?" or "Would you tell me where the men's room is?" or "What do you think the patient has got?" and as time goes by rehearse longer and more complicated sentences such as, for instance, "Do you know what the most impressive radiological finding of Chiari's is?" or "If I had known that the Chairman was not coming to the rounds, I would not have prepared the case so thoroughly".

Writing is the last step. In the recent past you would not have needed to write in English unless you were interested in publishing articles in foreign journals. You could even have spent a month abroad and not have had to write a single word other than your signature. Things have dramatically changed with the internet. Writing has become an absolute necessity for those who are in contact with foreign colleagues via e-mail. Being fluent writing e-mails will allow you to strengthen your links with other hospitals and colleagues by simply sending a few words periodically. The ability to communicate with foreign doctors will constitute a great competitive advantage. Once people are aware of this ability, you will soon be required to write messages and articles in English and, probably, you will be involved in more research projects than ever.

English spelling is not easy. There are a lot of double-consonant words and multiple possible pitfalls to avoid. Try to write words such as "14" or "40" and you will find the first difficulties. Is it "forteen" or "fourteen"? And what about 40?

Let me give you another piece of advice. Get used to writing in English on your computer. Select the English dictionary, and set it up so that every time you write a word incorrectly it will be underlined. Then punch the right button on your mouse and, instantaneously, a few alternative choices will appear on your screen, choose one and if it is correct go ahead. If you keep on doing this exercise, sooner or later your ability to write correctly will soon rise beyond what you could have ever imagined.

Some colleagues still think that medical English is so easy that it makes no sense to study it thoroughly. This is the same "oh-don't-worry case" that we see with English grammar. Here, you would hear people encouraging you with: "Don't worry, medical terminology is the same in all languages. It is all Latin. That's it. Humerus, tibia, radius …". But there is more to it than just implanting a Latin vowel or changing a few letters. This is good news because it makes our lives much more exciting. Life would be so dull and boring if translating medical knowledge from and into English was a simple addition or subtraction of letters. Talking about medical terminology can become a pleasurable pastime.

Unfortunately those who think that medical English is so easy do not give lectures abroad and, therefore, will never realize its real difficulty. Anyway, let us test our medical English level with these (easy?) exercises.

Exercise 1

Let us make a quick review of the carpal bones.

As everybody knows, or at least should know, the proximal row is made up of (from radial to ulnar) the naviculare, lunate, triquetrum, and pisiform bones.

Would you please read them in a correct manner?

It is likely you can read straightforwardly "naviculare", "lunate" and "pisiform", but I guess that reading "triquetrum" could be a little bit harder.

(Do not think that all Latin terms are as tricky as "triquetrum", but bear in mind that Latin can be an ally with regard to reading and an enemy in terms of pronunciation even for those health care professionals whose native language is based on Latin.)

Tip: When you look up a word in the dictionary, review not only its meaning but also both the phonetics and the spelling.

Exercice 2

What would you think if two radiologists are talking about the *PCP* interstitial pattern or that the most plausible cause of the pneumothorax was *LAM*?

- PCP stands for *Pneumocystis carinii* pneumonia.
- LAM stands for lymphangiomyomatosis.

Exercice 3

How would you start a formal letter to the Editor of a Medical Journal? Would it be acceptable to start "*Dear* Dr. Williams" even in the likely case that you do not know him at all?

- *Dear Dr. Williams* is an appropriate expression to start a formal letter.

And how would you finish it?

- *Sincerely yours* and *Faithfully yours* are the usual expressions to finish a formal letter. Generally, *Sincerely* should be used when you know the name of the person to whom you are writing, and *Faithfully* when you don't (i.e., starting with *Dear Sir*).

Exercice 4

Those non-fluent English speakers who often phone foreign colleagues are aware of the stressful situations they have had to overcome to get in touch with a colleague.

How should we start our conversation with Dr. Adams' secretary at 12:15 p.m. eastern time?

- Good afternoon. This is Dr. Adams' office.
- Good afternoon. This is Dr. Vida (instead of "Good morning. I am Dr. Vida"). May I talk to Dr. Adams?

Bear in mind that the usage of certain expressions can give the impression that you are fluent in English (probably more than you actually are) and Dr. Adams' secretary could overestimate your level and therefore speak more quickly. Do not hesitate to tell the secretary who is talking to you to speak up and slowly.

Exercise 5

Are you familiar with Latin plurals? We are sure that you can write *pneumothorax*, but what about its plural?

Is ultrasound (US) an effective *mean* of detecting gallbladder stones or is it an effective *means* of detecting them?

The right answers are:

* *Pneumothoraces.*
* US is an effective *means* of detecting gallbladder stones.

Exercise 6

Continue to revise simple conversational English questions. Choose the correct sentences from the following:

* The good news is that the problem can be solved.
* The good news are that the problem can be solved.

and

* The Chairman gave me some advice about the paper.
* The Chairman gave me some advices about the paper.

The right answers are:

* The good news is ...
* The Chairman gave me some advice...

Exercise 7

What does *ENT* stand for?
Ear, nose and throat.

Take into account that acronyms, especially if we try to translate them directly into English, can create strange, even embarrassing, situations. Whatever acronym is used in your native language to name temporomandibular-joint, forget it. In English it is "TMJ", and any other attempt could become a complete mess.

These exercises have been included to start an interesting game between you and this manual.

If you knew all the answers, this is obviously not the kind of book that you need because your level is above its goals. If you knew the answers to half the questions, this book could be very helpful and you will find some chapters below your level, so you can review known subjects, and some others above it, which will allow you to progress.

If you have barely been able to answer one or two questions, do not give up. The take-home message of this preliminary test could be that there is a lot of work to do and that probably medical English is not as easy as someone might have told you and, anyway, do not forget that virtually the only and more profitable way of correcting mistakes is by making them.

Fluency in a foreign language requires an important effort that lasts as long as your own life. The bad news is that even though you do your best, your English will always be improvable. On the other hand, the good news is that if you play this game you can take your progress for granted and your goals will be achieved, step by step, with effort but without sacrifice.

If you think that medical English is a vital tool in your professional career, go ahead. There is nothing more encouraging than your own commitment. If you belong to the overcrowded group that has thrown in the towel, please take your time to reconsider this subject. Your former approach to English was probably not the right one.

I deeply disagree with the teaching of English in many countries where medical English is not a crucial subject in medical school programs. The main problem in many educational systems is based upon the extraordinary amount of theoretical content to be studied, and English, in my opinion, is at the top of this educational disaster at least in my country. A high school student is supposed to be able to read Shakespeare plays and yet at the same time is barely able to decide whether to have meat or fish at a restaurant. I do believe that it is in English teaching that many educational systems have failed the most.

If you have not yet thrown in the towel but you are just on the verge of doing so, take this manual as your last opportunity and do not waste it. There is an "English boundary" at about age forty (did you spell it correctly on page 7?), although this imaginary line could be flexible depending on your motivation.

When you are starting your residency, English is still a failed subject but the towel has not been thrown in because an understanding of medical English is surely a worthy goal for anyone who wants to become a competitive physician. But during Residency there is a great obstacle to overcome, namely the calls. To study not only English but any other subject, residents must change calls and must attend classes when they are off-call. So, only a few of them can maintain the necessary motivation to keep on studying English, a subject that is not going to be evaluated, a subject that has no examinations at all.

A little bit later, as time goes by, residents get married and have children. Most of them thrive and become consultants, and English remains a failed subject; there is time left (or so they try to believe). Once they are in their forties, English remains a problem, and once a physician reaches this point, the chances are that English is going to be considered as a missing piece in their otherwise high standard of training.

The lack of notable confidence in English is responsible for a great number of missed chances in our career. When either a resident or an attending physician is considering going abroad to an American or British hospital to do some research work there are two main barriers to be overcome. The first, and most important one, is English. In many countries, no English examinations need to be taken after high school years, and time has eroded the scarce, if any, remaining concepts learnt during our school days. The second barrier is economic, but this is undoubtedly less important than knowledge of English. I have met many residents whose economic situation was extremely difficult in American hospitals. Their English was reasonably fluent and their economic situation did not undermine their training. Indeed, they probably were more engaged in their academic tasks because they had no money to spend outside the hospital. On the contrary, I have not met any non-English-speaking foreign resident in the US.

Once you realize that confidence in your medical English is the only way to receive a state-of-the-art training in your medical specialty, your motivation will help you overcome all the obstacles and the possibilities open to you will grow without any geographical boundaries.

Don't you think it is time to overcome this overwhelming enemy? Give it a try and do not forget that studying English is like a diet – both are a question of lifestyle – endless tasks to be performed for the rest of our lives and, therefore, these tasks must be bearable unless we give up and all our efforts become unproductive.

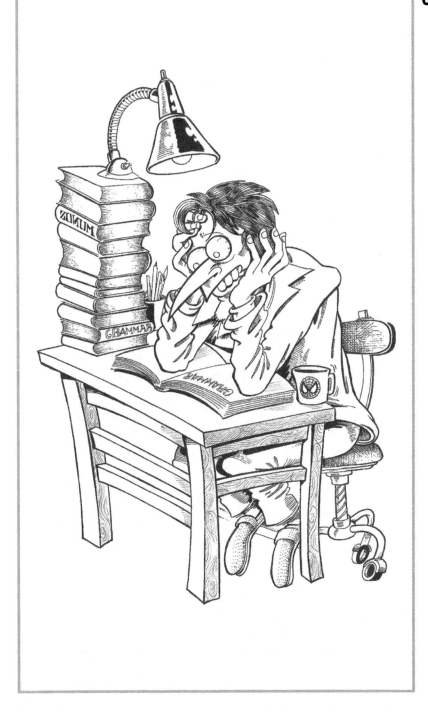

Unit II Grammar in Use

Introduction

In this unit we review some of the most important English grammatical structures using as examples normal sentences in medical environments. We could say, to summarize, that we have replaced the classical sentence of old English manuals "my tailor is rich" by expressions such as "the first year resident is on call today". Without a sound grammatical background it is not possible to speak correctly just as without a profound knowledge of anatomy it should not be possible to report on radiological examinations. The tendency to skip both grammar and anatomy, considered by many as simple preliminary issues, has had deleterious effects on the learning of English and medicine.

Tenses

Talking About the Present

Present continuous

Present continuous shows an action that is happening in the present time at or around the moment of speaking.

> **FORM**
>
> Present simple of the verb *to be* + gerund of the verb: am/are/is -ing.
>
> Study this example:
>
> It is 7.00 in the morning. Dr. Smith is in his new car on his way to the hospital.
>
> So: He *is driving* to the hospital. He is driving to the hospital means that he is driving now, at the time of speaking.

To talk about:

- Something that is happening at the time of speaking (i.e., now):
  - Dr. Smith *is going* to the operating room.
  - Dr. Smith's colleague *is operating on* an acute cholecystitis.

- Something that is happening around or close to the time of speaking, but not necessarily exactly at the time of speaking:
  - John and Rachel are residents of neurology and they are having a sandwich in the cafeteria. John says:
    "I *am writing* an interesting article on multiple sclerosis. I'll lend it to you when I've finished it".
    As you can see John is not writing the article at the time of speaking. He means that he has begun to write the article but has not finished it yet. He is in the middle of writing it.

- Something that is happening for a limited period of time around the present (e.g. today, this week, this season, this year...):
  - Our residents *are working* hard this term.

- Changing situations:
  - The patient *is getting* better with the new treatment.
  - His blood pressure *is rising* very fast.

- Temporary situations:
  - I *am living* with other residents until I can buy my own apartment.

Present continuous with a future meaning

In the following examples doing these things is already arranged.

- To talk about what you have arranged to do in the near future (personal arrangements).
  - We *are stenting* a renal artery on Monday.
  - I *am having* dinner with a medical representative tomorrow.

We can also use the form *going to* in these sentences, but it is less natural when you talk about arrangements.
We do not use the simple present or *will* for personal arrangements.

Simple present

Simple present shows an action that happens again and again (repeated action) in the present time, but not necessarily at the time of speaking.

FORM

The simple present has the following forms:

- Affirmative (remember to add -s or -es to the third person singular)
- Negative
  - I/we/you/they don't...
  - He/she/it doesn't...

- Interrogative
  - Do I/we/you/they...?
  - Does he/she/it...?

Study this example:

Dr. Allan is the chairman of the radiology department. He is in Greece on an international course.

So: He *is not running* the radiology department now (because he is in Greece), but *he runs* the radiology department.

USES

- To talk about something that happens all the time or repeatedly or something that is true in general. Here it is not important whether the action is happening at the time of speaking:
  - I *do* interventional radiology.
  - Nurses *take* care of patients.
  - Cigarettes *cause* lung cancer.

- To say how often we do things:
  - I *begin* to operate at 8.30 every morning.
  - Dr. Taylor *does* angioplasty two evenings a week.
  - How often *do you go* to the cardiologist? Once a month.

- For a permanent situation (a situation that stays the same for a long time):
  - I *work* as an endocrinologist in the diabetes program of our hospital. I have been working there for ten years.

- Some verbs are used only in simple tenses. These verbs are verbs of thinking or mental activity, feeling, possession and perception, and reporting verbs. We often use *can* instead of the present tense with verbs of perception:
  - I now *understand* why the patient is in such a bad condition.
  - I *can see* the solution to your problem now.

- The simple present is often used with adverbs of frequency such as always, often, sometimes, rarely, never, every week, and twice a year:
  - The chairman *is always* working.

<table>
<tr><td>USES</td><td>

- Simple present with a future meaning. We use it to talk about timetables, schedules ...:
  - What time does Ross' operation conference start? It *starts* tomorrow at 9.30.
</td></tr>
</table>

Talking About the Future

Going To

<table>
<tr><td>USES</td><td>

- To say what we have already decided to do or what we intend to do in the future (do not use *will* in this situation):
  - I *am going to* attend the 20th International Congress of Cardiology next month.
  - There is a CT course in Boston next fall. *Are you going to* attend it?

- To say what someone has arranged to do (personal arrangements), but remember that we prefer to use the present continuous because it sounds more natural:
  - What time *are you meeting* the vice chairman?

- To say what we think will happen (making predictions):
  - The patient is looking terrible. I think he *is going to* die soon.

- If we want to say what someone intended to do in the past but did not do, we use *was/were going to*:
  - He *was going to* do a CT on the patient but changed his mind.

- To talk about past predictions we use *was/were going to*:
  - She *was going to* become a good surgeon.
</td></tr>
</table>

Simple Future (Will)

<table>
<tr><td>FORM</td><td>

I/We *will* or *shall* (*will* is more common than *shall*. Shall is often used in questions to make offers and suggestions): *Shall* we go to the symposium next week?
You/he/she/it/they *will*.
Negative: *shan't, won't*.
</td></tr>
</table>

USES

- We use *it* when we decide to do something at the time of speaking (remember that in this situation, you cannot use the simple present):
  - Have you called the cardiologist?
  - No, I haven't had time to do it.
  - OK, don't worry, I *will* do it.

- When offering, agreeing, refusing and promising to do something, or when asking someone to do something:
  - That case looks difficult for you. I *will* help you.
  - Can I have the book I lent you last week back? Of course. I *will* give it back to you tomorrow.
  - Don't ask to use his stethoscope. He *won't* lend it to you.
  - I promise I *will* send you a copy of the latest article on AIDS as soon as I get it.
  - *Will* you help me with this patient, please?

You do not use *will* to say what someone has already decided to do or arranged to do (remember that in this situation we use *going to* or the present continuous):

- To predict a future happening or a future situation:
  - Medicine *will* be very different in a hundred years time.
  - Neurology *won't* be the same in the next two decades.

Remember that if there is something in the present situation that shows us what will happen in the future (near future) we use *going to* instead of *will*:

- With expressions such as: *probably, I am sure, I bet, I think, I suppose, I guess*:
  - I *will* probably attend the European Congress.
  - You should listen to Dr. Higgins giving a conference. I am sure you *will* love it.
  - I bet the patient *will* recover satisfactorily.
  - I guess I *will* see you in the next annual meeting.

Future Continuous

FORM

Will be + gerund of the verb.

<table>
<tr><td>USES</td><td>

● To say that we will be in the middle of something at a certain time in the future:
  - This time tomorrow morning I *will* be attending the conference about drugs and the CNS.

● To talk about things that are already planned or decided (similar to the present continuous with a future meaning):
  - We can't meet this evening. I *will* be operating on the patient we talked about.

● To ask about people's plans, especially when we want something or want someone to do something (interrogative form):
  - *Will* you be attending to my patients this evening?

</td></tr>
</table>

Future Perfect

FORM	*Will have* + past participle of the verb.

USES	● To say that something will already have happened before a certain time in the future: - I think the liver *will* already *have arrived* by the time we begin the transplantation. - Next spring I *will have been* working for 25 years in this hospital.

Talking About the Past

Simple Past

FORM	The simple past has the following forms: ● Affirmative: - The past of the regular verbs is formed by adding -ed to the infinitive. - The past of the irregular verbs has its own form. ● Negative: - *Did/didn't* + the base form of the verb. ● Questions: - *Did I/you/...* + the base form of the verb

- To talk about actions or situations in the past (they have already finished):
  - I *enjoyed* the resident's party very much.
  - When I worked as a resident in Madrid, I *lived* in a small apartment.

- To say that one thing happened after another:
  - Yesterday we *had* a terrible duty. We *operated on* five patients and then we *did* a kidney transplantation.

- To ask or say *when* or *what time* something happened:
  - When were you *operated on* last time?

- To tell a story and to talk about happenings and actions that are not connected with the present (historical events):
  - Roentgen *discovered* X-rays.

Past Continuous

FORM

Was/were + gerund of the verb.

USES

- To say that someone was in the middle of doing something at a certain time. The action or situation had already started before this time but hadn't finished:
  - This time last year I *was writing* an article on lipid metabolism.

Notice that the past continuous does not tell us whether an action was finished or not. Perhaps it was, perhaps it was not.

- To describe a scene:
  - A lot of patients *were waiting* in the corridor.

Present Perfect

FORM

Have/has + past participle of the verb.

USES

- To talk about the present result of a past action.
- To talk about a recent happening.

In the latter situation you can use the present perfect with the following particles:

- *Just* (i.e., a short time ago): to say something has happened a short time ago:
  - Dr. Ho *has just arrived* at the hospital.

- *Already*: to say something has happened sooner than expected:
  - The second-year resident *has already finished* her presentation.

Remember that to talk about a recent happening we can also use the simple past:

- A period of time that continues up to the present (an unfinished period of time):
  - We use the expressions: *today, this morning, this evening, this week…*
  - We often use *ever* and *never*.

- Something that we are expecting. In this situation we use *yet* to show that the speaker is expecting something to happen, but only in questions and negative sentences:
  - Dr. Goyen *has not arrived yet.*
  We can also use *yet* with the simple past:
  - Dr. Goyen *did not arrive yet.*

- Something you have never done or something you have not done during a period of time that continues up to the present:
  - I *have not reported* a CT scan since I was a resident.

- How much we have done, how many things we have done or how many times we have done something:
  - I *have attended* to ten patients today.
  - Dr. Concepcion *has operated* on four hearts this weekend.

- Situations that exist for a long time, especially if we say *always*. In this case the situation still exists now:
  - Dr. Suárez de Lezo *has always worked* very hard.
  - Dr. Pera *has always been* a very talented surgeon.

We also use the present perfect with these expressions:

- Superlative: *It is the most …*:
  - It is the most interesting case that I *have ever seen.*

- *The first (second, third…) time …*:
  - This is the first time that I *have seen* a patient with Wilson's disease.

Present Perfect Continuous

Shows an action that began in the past and has gone on up to the present time.

FORM	*Have/has been* + gerund.

USES	• To talk about an action that began in the past and has recently stopped or just stopped: – You look tired. *Have you been studying?* – Yes, *I have been studying* the Pancoast case. • To ask or say how long something has been happening. In this case the action or situation began in the past and is still happening or has just stopped. – Dr. Sancho and Dr. Martos *have been working* in the project from its inception.

We use the following particles:

- *How long...?* (to ask how long).

- *For, since* (to say how long):
  - *How long* have you been working as a family doctor?
  - I have been working *for* ten years.
  - I have been working very hard *since* I got this post.

- *For* (to say how long as a period of time):
  - I have been studying MR imaging *for* three months.
  Do not use *for* in expressions with *all*:
  I have worked as a doctor *all* my life (not "*for all* my life").

- *Since* (to say the beginning of a period):
  - I have been teaching anatomy *since* 1980.

In the present perfect continuous the important thing is the action itself and it does not matter whether the action is finished or not. The action can be finished (just finished) or not (still happening).

In the present perfect the important thing is the result of the action and not the action itself. The action is completely finished.

Past Perfect

Shows an action that happened in the past before another past action. It is the past of the present perfect.

FORM	*Had* + past participle of the verb.

USES	• To say that something had already happened before something else happened: – When I arrived at the meeting, the chairman *had* already *begun* his presentation.

Past Perfect Continuous

Shows an action that began in the past and went on up to a time in the past. It is the past of the present perfect continuous.

	Had been + gerund of the verb.

USES	• To say how long something had been happening before something else happened: – She *had been working* as an endocrinologist for forty years before she was awarded the Nobel prize.

Subjunctive

Imagine this situation:
• The surgeon says to the radiologist, "Why don't you do a CT scan to the patient with an acute abdominal pain?"
• The surgeon proposes (that) the radiologist do a CT scan to the patient with an acute abdominal pain.

The subjunctive is formed always with the base form of the verb (the infinitive without to):
• I suggest (that) you *work* harder.
• She recommended (that) he *give up* drinking alcohol.

- He insisted (that) she *operate on* the patient as soon as possible.
- He demanded (that) the nurse *treat him* more politely.

Note that the subjunctive of the verb *to be* is usually passive:
- He insisted (that) the patient *be admitted* immediately.

You can use the subjunctive after:
- Propose
- Suggest
- Recommend
- Insist
- Demand

You can use the subjunctive for the past, present or future:
- He *suggested* (that) the resident *change* the treatment.
- He *recommends* (that) his patients *give up* smoking.
  Should is sometimes used instead of the subjunctive:
- The doctor recommended that *I should give up* smoking for the rest of my life.

Wish, If Only, Would

Wish

- *Wish* + simple past. To say that we regret something (i.e., that something is not as we would like it to be) in the present:
  - *I wish I were* not on call tomorrow (but I am on call tomorrow).

- *Wish* + past perfect. To say that we regret something that happened or didn't happen in the past:
  - *I wish he hadn't treated* the patient's family so badly (but he treated the patient's family badly).

- *Wish* + *would* + infinitive without *to* when we want something to happen or change or somebody to do something:
  - *I wish you wouldn't take* the clinical histories so fast (note that the speaker is complaining about the present situation or the way people do things).

If Only
If only can be used in exactly the same way as *wish*. It has the same meaning as *wish* but is more dramatic:
- *If only* + past simple (expresses regret in the present):
  - *If only I were not* on call tomorrow.

- *If only* + past perfect (expresses regret in the past):
  - *If only he hadn't treated* the patient's family so badly.

After *wish* and *if only* we use *were* (with *I, he, she, it*) instead of *was*, and we do not normally use *would*, although sometimes it is possible, or *would have*.

When referring to the present or future, *wish* and *if only* are followed by a past tense, and when referring to the past by a past perfect tense.

Would
Would is used:

- As a modal verb in offers, invitations and requests (i.e., to ask someone to do something):
  - *Would* you help me to write an article on long-term prognosis of patients with myocardial infarction? (request).
  - *Would* you like to come to the residents' party tonight? (offer and invitation).

- After *wish*.

- In *if* sentences (see conditional).

- Sometimes as the past of *will* (in reported speech):
  - Dr. Smith: I will operate on your ankle next week.
  - Patient: The doctor said that he *would* operate on me next week.

- When you remember things that often happened (similar to *used to*):
  - When we were residents, we used to prepare the clinical cases together.
  - When we were residents, we *would* prepare the clinical cases together.

Modal Verbs

A modal verb has always the same form.

There is no *-s* ending in the third person singular, no *-ing* form and no *-ed* form.

After a modal verb we use the infinitive without *to* (i.e., the base form of the verb).

These are the English modal verbs:

- *Can* (past form is *could*)
- *Could* (also a modal with its own meaning)
- *May* (past form is *might*)
- *Might* (also a modal with its own meaning)
- *Will*
- *Would*
- *Shall*
- *Should*

- *Ought to*
- *Must*
- *Need*
- *Dare*

We use modal verbs to talk about:

- Ability
- Necessity
- Possibility
- Certainty
- Permission
- Obligation

Expressing Ability

To express ability we can use:

- *Can* (only in the present tense)
- *Could* (only in the past tense)
- *Be able to* (in all tenses)

Ability in the Present

Can (more usual) or *am/is/are able to* (less usual):

- Dr. Williams *can* operate on extremely difficult hepatic tumors.
- Dr. Ross *is able to* operate on colonic tumors.
- *Can* you speak medical English? Yes, I *can*.
- *Are you able to* speak medical English? Yes, I am.

Ability in the Past

Could (past form of *can*) or *was/were able to*.

We use *could* to say that someone had the *general* ability to do something:

- When I was a resident I *could* speak German

We use *was/were able to* to say that someone managed to do something in one particular situation (*specific* ability to do something):

- When I was a resident I *was able to* do fifteen duties in one month.

Managed to can replace *was able to*:

- When I was a resident I *managed to* do fifteen duties in one month

We use *could have* to say that we had the ability to do something but we didn't do it:

● He *could have* been a surgeon but he became a pediatrician instead.

Sometimes we use *could* to talk about ability in a situation which we are imagining. Here *could = would be able to*:

● I couldn't do your job. I'm not clever enough.

We use *will be able to* to talk about ability with a future meaning:

● If you keep on studying medical English you *will be able to* write articles very soon.

Expressing Necessity

Necessity means that you cannot avoid doing something.

To say that it is necessary to do something we can use *must* or *have to*:

● Necessity in the present: *must, have/has to*.
● Necessity in the past: *had to*.
● Necessity in the future: *must* or *will have to*.

Notice that to express necessity in the past we do not use *must*.

There are some differences between *must* and *have to*:

● We use *must* when the speaker is expressing personal feelings or authority, saying what he or she thinks is necessary:
  – Your cough is terrible. You *must* give up smoking

● We use *have to* when the speaker is not expressing personal feelings or authority. The speaker is just giving facts or expressing the authority of another person (external authority), often a law or a rule:
  – All citizens *have to* pay the Social Security Tax.

If we want to express that there is a necessity to avoid doing something, we use *mustn't* (i.e., *not allowed to*):

● You *mustn't* drink alcohol while taking these tablets.

Expressing No Necessity

To express that there is no necessity we can use the negative forms of *need* or *have to*:

- No necessity in the present: *needn't* or *don't/doesn't have to.*
- No necessity in the past: *didn't need, didn't have to.*
- No necessity in the future: *won't have to.*

Notice that "there is no necessity to do something" is completely different from "there is a necessity not to do something".

In conclusion, we use *mustn't* when we are not allowed to do something or when there is a necessity not to do it, and we use the negative form of *have to* or *needn't* when there is no necessity to do something but we can do it if we want to:

- The doctor says *I mustn't* get overtired but *I needn't* stay in bed.
- The doctor says *I mustn't* get overtired but *I don't have to* stay in bed.

Expressing Possibility

To express possibility we can use *can, could, may* or *might* (from more to less certainty: can → may → might → could).

Possibility in the Present

To say that something is possible we use *can, may, might, could*:
- Food with plenty of fiber *can* be very good for you (high level of certainty).
- Eating more fiber *may* actually help you to slim (moderate to high level of certainty).
- Eating healthy food *might* help you to lose 10 pounds (moderate to low level of certainty).
- Eating vegetables *could* help you to lose 20 pounds (low level of certainty).

Possibility in the Past

To say that something was possible in the past we use *may have, might have, could have*:

- The patient *might have* survived if the ambulance had arrived earlier.

Could have is also used to say that something was a possibility or opportunity but it didn't happen:

- You were lucky to be treated with that antibiotic; if not, you *could have* died.

I *couldn't have* done something (i.e., I wouldn't have been able to do it if I had wanted or tried to do it):

* She *couldn't have* seen him anyway because she was in bed.

Possibility in the Future

To talk about possible future actions or happenings we use *may, might, could* (especially in suggestions):

* I don't know where to do my last six months of residence. I *may/might* go to the States.
* We *could* meet later in the hospital to review some cases, couldn't we?

When we are talking about possible future plans we can also use the continuous form *may/might/could be* + *-ing* form:

* I *could be going* to the RSNA Congress next fall.

Expressing Certainty

To say we are sure that something is true we use *must*:

* You have been operating all night. You *must* be tired (i.e., I am sure that you are tired).

To say that we think something is impossible we use *can't*:

* According to his clinical situation, that diagnosis *can't* be true (i.e., It is impossible that that diagnosis be true *or* I am sure that that diagnosis is not true).

For past situations we use *must have* and *can't have*. We can also use *couldn't have* instead of *can't have*:

* Taking into consideration the situation, the family of the patient *couldn't have* asked for more.

Remember that to express certainty we can also use *will*:

* If his heart rate does not decrease, the patient *will* die.

Expressing Permission

To talk about permission we can use *can, may* (more formal than *can*) or *be allowed to.*

Permission in the Present

Can, may or *am/is/are allowed to*:

- You *can* smoke if you like.
- You *are allowed to* smoke.
- You *may* attend the Congress.

Permission in the Past

Was/were allowed to:

- *Were you allowed to* go in the ICU without surgical scrubs?

Permission in the Future

Will be allowed to:

- *I will be allowed to* leave the hospital when my duty is off.

To ask for permission we use *can, may, could* or *might* (from less to more formal) but not *be allowed to*:

- Hi Derek, *can* I borrow your stethoscope? (if you are asking for a friend's stethoscope).
- Dr. Putin, *may* I borrow your stethoscope? (if you are talking to an acquaintance).
- *Could* I use your stethoscope, Dr. Ho? (if you are talking to a colleague you do not know at all).
- *Might* I use your stethoscope, Dr. De Roos? (if you are asking for the chairman's stethoscope).

Expressing Obligation or Giving Advice

Obligation means that something is the right thing to do.

When we want to say what we think is a good thing to do or the right thing to do we use *should* or *ought to* (a little stronger than *should*).

Should and *ought to* can be used for giving advice:

- You *ought* to sleep.
- You *should* work out.
- You *ought* to give up smoking.
- *Ought* he to see a doctor? Yes, I think he ought to.
- *Should* he see a doctor? Yes, I think he should.

Conditionals

Conditional sentences have two parts:

1. "If-clause"
2. Main clause

In the sentence "If I were you I would go to the annual meeting of orthopedics", "If I were you" is the if-clause, and "I would go to the annual meeting of orthopedics" is the main clause.

The if-clause can come before or after the main clause. We often put a comma when the if-clause comes first.

Main Types of Conditional Sentences

Type 0

To talk about things that always are true (general truths).

FORMS	*If* + simple present + simple present: • *If* you inject insulin to a person, the glucose blood level decreases. • *If* you drink too much alcohol, you get a sore head. • *If* you take drugs habitually, you become addicted.

Note that the examples above refer to things that are normally true. They make no reference to the future; they represent a present simple concept. This is the basic (or classic) form of the conditional type 0.

There are possible variations of this form. In the if-clause and in the main clause we can use the present continuous, present perfect simple or present perfect continuous instead of the present simple. In the main clause we can also use the imperative instead of the present simple:

• Residents only get a certificate *if* they have attended the course regularly.

So the type 0 form can be reduced to:

• *If* + present form + present form or imperative.

Present forms include the present simple, present continuous, present perfect simple, and present perfect continuous.

Type 1

To talk about future situations that the speaker thinks are likely to happen (the speaker is thinking about a real possibility in the future).

> **FORM**
>
> *If* + simple present + future simple (*will*):
>
> - *If* I find something new about the treatment of myocardial infarction, I will tell you.
> - *If* we can analyze genomes, we will be able to infer laws and principles about them.

These examples refer to future things that are possible and it is quite probable that they will happen. This is the basic (or classic) form of the conditional type 1.

There are possible variations of the basic form. In the if-clause we can use the present continuous, the present perfect or the present perfect continuous instead of the present simple. In the main clause we can use future continuous, future perfect simple or future perfect continuous instead of the future simple. Modals such as *can*, *may* or *might* are also possible.

So the form of type 1 can be reduced to:

- *If* + present form + future form

Future forms include the future simple, future continuous, future perfect simple, and future perfect continuous.

Type 2

To talk about future situations that the speaker thinks are possible but not probable (the speaker is imagining a possible future situation) or to talk about unreal situations in the present.

> **FORM**
>
> *If* + simple past + conditional (*would*):
>
> - Peter, *if* you *studied* harder, you *would* be better prepared for doing your job.

The above sentence tells us that Peter is supposed not to be studying hard.

- *If* I *were* you, I *would* go to the Annual Meeting of Cardiology (but I am not you).

- *If* I *were* a resident again I *would* go to Harvard Medical School for a whole year to complete my training period (but I am not a resident).

There are possible variations of the basic form. In the if-clause we can use the past continuous instead the past simple. In the main clause we can use *could* or *might* instead of *would*.

So the form of type 2 can be reduced to:

- *If* + past simple or continuous + *would, could* or *might*.

Type 3

To talk about past situations that didn't happen (impossible actions in the past).

> **FORM**
>
> *If* + past perfect + perfect conditional (*would have*):
>
> - *If* I *had known* the patient's diagnosis, *I would* probably *have* saved his life.

As you can see, we are talking about the past. The real situation is that I didn't know the patient's diagnosis so that I couldn't save his life.

This is the basic (or classic) form of the third type of conditional. There are possible variations. In the if-clause we can use the past perfect continuous instead of the past perfect simple. In the main clause we can use the continuous form of the perfect conditional instead of the perfect conditional simple. *Would probably, could* or *might* instead of *would* are also possible (when we are not sure about something).

In Case

"The surgeon wears two pairs of latex gloves during an operation in case one of them tears." *In case one of them tears* because it is possible that one of them tears during the operation (in the future).

Note that we don't use *will* after *in case*. We use a present tense after *in case* when we are talking about the future.

In case is not the same as *if*. Compare these sentences:

- We'll buy some more food and drink *if* the new residents come to our department's party. (Perhaps the new residents will come to our party. If they come, we will buy some more food and drink; if they don't come, we won't.)

- We will buy some food and drink *in case* the new residents come to our department's party. (Perhaps the new residents will come to our department's party. We will buy some more food and drink whether they come or not.)

We can also use *in case* to say why someone did something in the past:

- He rang the bell again *in case* the nurse hadn't heard it the first time. (Because it was possible that the nurse hadn't heard it the first time.)

In case of (= if there is):

- *In case of* fire, use the emergency exits to leave the hospital. (If there is a fire, use the emergency exits to leave the hospital.)

Unless

"Don't take these pills *unless* you are extremely anxious." (Don't take these pills except if you are extremely anxious.) This sentence means that you can take the pills only if you are extremely anxious.

We use *unless* to make an exception to something we say. In the example above the exception is *you are extremely anxious.*

We often use *unless* in warnings:

- Unless you send the application form today, you won't be accepted in the next National Congress of Rheumatology.

It is also possible to use *if* in a negative sentence instead of *unless*:

- Don't take those pills *if you aren't* extremely anxious.
- *If you don't send* the application form today, you won't be accepted in the next Congress of Rheumatology.

As Long As, Provided (That), Providing (That)

These expressions mean *but only if*:

- You can use my new pen to take the clinical history *as long as* you write carefully (i.e., *but only if* you write carefully).
- Going by car to the hospital is convenient *provided (that)* you have somewhere to park (i.e., *but only if* you have somewhere to park).
- *Providing (that)* she studies the clinical cases, she will deliver a bright presentation.

Passive Voice

Study these examples:

- The first case of AIDS was described in 1984 (passive sentence).
- Someone described the first case of AIDS in 1984 (active sentence).

Both sentences are correct and mean the same. They are two different ways of saying the same thing but in the passive sentence we try to make the object of the active sentence (the first case of AIDS) more important by putting it at the beginning. So, we prefer to use the passive when it is not that important who or what did the action. In the example above, it is not so important (or not known) who described the first case of AIDS.

Active sentence:

- Fleming (subject) discovered (active verb) penicillin (object) in 1950.

Passive sentence:

- Penicillin (subject) was discovered (passive verb) by Fleming (agent) in 1950.

The passive verb is formed by putting the verb *to be* into the same tense as the active verb and adding the past participle of the active verb:

- Discovered (active verb) – was discovered (*be* + past participle of the active verb).

The object of an active verb becomes the subject of the passive verb (*penicillin*). The subject of an active verb becomes the agent of the passive verb (*Fleming*). We can leave out the agent if it is not important to mention it or we don't know it. If we want to mention it, we will put it at the end of the sentence preceded by the particle *by* (... *by Fleming*).

Some sentences have two objects, indirect and direct. In these sentences the passive subject can be either the direct object or the indirect object of the active sentence:

- The doctor gave the patient a new treatment.

There are two possibilities:

- A new treatment was given to the patient.
- The patient was given a new treatment.

Passive Forms of Present and Past Tenses

Simple present

Active:
- Doctors review the most interesting cases in the clinical session every day.

Passive:
- The most interesting cases are reviewed every day in the clinical session.

Simple past

Active:
- The nurse checked the blood pressure of the patient before the operation.

Passive:
- The blood pressure of the patient was checked before the operation.

Present continuous

Active:
- The surgeons are operating on an old woman right now.

Passive:
- An old woman is being operated on right now.

Past continuous

Active:
- They were carrying the injured person to the hospital.

Passive:
- The injured person was being carried to the hospital.

Present perfect

Active:
- The doctor has attended to ten patients this morning.

Passive:
- Ten patients have been attended to this morning.

Past perfect

Active:
- They had sent the CT films before the operation started.

Passive:
- The CT films had been sent before the operation started.

In sentences of the type "people say/consider/know/think/believe/expect/understand... that...", such as *Doctors consider that AIDS is a fatal disease,* we have two possible passive forms:

- AIDS is considered to be a fatal disease.
- It is considered that AIDS is a fatal disease.

Have/Get Something Done

FORM	*Have/get* + object + past participle.

Get is a little more informal than *have*, and it is often used in informal spoken English:

- You should *get* your eyes tested.
- You should *have* your eyes tested.

When we want to say that we don't do something by ourselves and we arrange for someone to do it for us, we use the expression *have something done*:

- He had his gallbladder removed in order to prevent an acute cholecystitis.

Sometimes the expression *have something done* has a different meaning:

- John had his knee broken playing a football match.

It is obvious that this doesn't mean that he arranged for somebody to break his knee. With this meaning, we use *have something done* to say that something (often something not nice) happened to someone.

Supposed To

Supposed to can be used in the following ways:

- Can be used like *said to*:
  - The chairman is supposed to be the one who runs the Department.

- To say what is planned or arranged (and this is often different from what really happens):
  - The fourth year resident is supposed to attend to this patient.

- To say what is not allowed or not advisable:
  - She was not supposed to be on call yesterday.

Reported Speech

Imagine that you want to tell someone else what the patient said. You can either repeat the patient's words or use reported speech.

The reporting verb (*said* in the examples below) can come before or after the reported clause (*there was a conference about cardiac MR that evening*), but it usually comes before the reported clause. When the reporting verb comes before, we can use *that* to introduce the reported clause or we can leave it out (leaving it out is more informal). When the reporting verb comes after, we cannot use *that* to introduce the reported clause.

The reporting verb can report statements and thoughts, questions, orders, and requests.

Reporting in the Present

When the reporting verb is in the present tense, it isn't necessary to change the tense of the verb:

- "I'll help you guys to operate on this knee", he says.
- He says (that) he will help us to operate on this knee.
- "The vertebroplasty will take place this morning", he says.
- He says (that) the vertebroplasty will take place this morning.

Reporting in the Past

When the reporting verb is in the past tense, the verb in direct speech usually changes in the following ways:

- Simple present changes to simple past.
- Present continuous changes to past continuous.
- Simple past changes to past perfect.
- Past continuous changes to past perfect continuous.
- Present perfect changes to past perfect.
- Present perfect continuous changes to past perfect continuous.
- Past perfect stays the same.
- Future changes to conditional.

- Future continuous changes to conditional continuous.
- Future perfect changes to conditional perfect.
- Conditional stays the same.
- Present forms of modal verbs stay the same.
- Past forms of modal verbs stay the same.

Pronouns, adjectives and adverbs also change. Here are some examples:

- First person singular changes to third person singular.
- Second person singular changes to first person singular.
- First person plural changes to third person plural.
- Second person plural changes to first person plural.
- Third person singular changes to third person plural.
- Now changes to then.
- Today changes to that day.
- Tomorrow changes to the day after.
- Yesterday changes to the day before.
- This changes to that.
- Here changes to there.
- Ago changes to before.

It is not always necessary to change the verb when you use reported speech. If you are reporting something and you feel that it is still true, you do not need to change the tense of the verb, but if you want you can do it:

- The treatment of choice of HZV infections is acyclovir.
- He said (that) the treatment of choice of HZV infections is acyclovir.

or

- He said (that) the treatment of choice of HZV infections was acyclovir.

Reporting Questions

Yes and No Questions

We use *whether* or *if*:

- Do you smoke or drink any alcohol?
  - The doctor asked if I smoked or drank any alcohol.

- Have you had any diarrhea?
  - The doctor asked me whether I had had any diarrhea or not.

- Are you taking any pills or medicines at the moment?
  - The doctor asked me if I was taking any pills or medicines at that moment.

Wh... Questions

We use the same question word as in the *wh...* question:

- What do you mean by saying you are feeling under the weather?
  - The doctor asked me what I meant by saying I was feeling under the weather.
- Why do you think you feel under the weather?
  - The doctor asked me why I thought I felt under the weather
- When do you feel under the weather?
  - The doctor asked me when I felt under the weather.
- How often do you have headaches?
  - The doctor asked how often I had headaches.

Reported Questions

Reported questions have the following characteristics:
1. The word order is different from the original question. The verb follows the subject as in an ordinary statement.
2. The auxiliary verb *do* is not used.
3. There is no question mark.
4. The verb changes in the same way as in direct speech.

Study the following examples:

- How old are you?
  - The doctor asked me how old I was.
- Do you smoke?
  - The doctor asked me if I smoked.

Reporting Orders and Requests

FORM	*Tell* (pronoun) + object (indirect) + infinitive:

	• Take the pills before meals.
	    – The doctor told me to take the pills before meals.
	
	 • You mustn't smoke.
	    – The doctor told me not to smoke.

Reporting Suggestions and Advice

Suggestions and advice are reported in the following forms:

- Suggestions
  - Why don't we operate on that patient this evening?
  - The surgeon suggested operating on that patient that evening.

- Advice
  - You had better stay in bed.
  - The doctor advised me to stay in bed.

Questions

In sentences with *to be*, *to have* (in its auxiliary form) and modal verbs, we usually make questions by changing the word order:

- Affirmative
  - You are a medical doctor.
  - Interrogative: Are you a medical doctor?

- Negative
  - You are not a medical doctor.
  - Interrogative: Aren't you a medical doctor?

In simple present questions we use *do/does*:

- His stomach hurts.
- Does his stomach hurt?

In simple past questions we use *did*:

- The nurse arrived on time.
- Did the nurse arrive on time?

If *who/what/which* is the subject of the sentence we do not use *do*:

- Someone paged Dr. W.
- Who paged Dr. W?

If *who/what/which* is the object of the sentence we use *did*:

- Dr. W. paged someone.
- Who did Dr. W. page?

When we ask somebody and begin the question with *Do you know...* or *Could you tell me...*, the rest of the question maintains the affirmative sentence's word order:

- Where is the cafeteria?

but

- Do you know where the cafeteria is?
- Where is the library?

but

- Could you tell me where the library is?

Reported questions also maintain the affirmative sentence's word order:

- Dr. Wilson asked: How are you?

but

- Dr. Wilson asked me how I was.

Short answers are possible in questions where *be, do, can, have* and *might* are auxiliary verbs:

- Do you smoke? Yes, I do.
- Did you smoke? No, I didn't.
- Can you walk? Yes, I can.

We also use auxiliary verbs with *so* (affirmative) and *neither* or *nor* (negative) changing the word order:

- I am feeling tired. So am I.
- I can't remember the disease name. Neither can I.
- Is he going to pass the boards? I think so.
- Will you be on call tomorrow? I guess not.
- Will you be off call the day after tomorrow? I hope so.
- Has the Chairman been invited to the party? I'm afraid so.

Tag questions. We use a positive tag question with a negative sentence and vice versa:

- The first year resident isn't feeling very well today, is she?
- You are working late at the lab, aren't you?

After *let's* the tag question is *shall we*?

- Let's read a couple of articles, shall we?

After the imperative, the tag question is *will you*?

- Close the door, will you?

Infinitive/-*Ing*

Verb + -*Ing*

There are certain verbs that are usually used in the structure verb + -*ing* when followed by another verb:

- *Stop*: Please *stop talking*.
- *Finish*: *I've finished translating* the article.
- *Enjoy*: I *enjoy talking* to patients while I'm in the ward.
- *Mind*: I *don't mind being* told what to do.
- *Suggest*: Dr. Knight *suggested going* to the OT and trying to operate on the aneurysm.
- *Dislike*: She *dislikes going* out late after a night on-call.
- *Imagine*: I *can't imagine you operating*. You told me you hate blood.
- *Regret*: *The regrets having gone* two minutes before his patient had seizures.
- *Admit*: The resident *admitted forgetting* to change Mr. Smith's treatment.
- *Consider*: Have you *considered finishing* your residence in the USA?

Other verbs that follow this structure are: *avoid, deny, involve, practice, miss, postpone,* and *risk*.

The following expressions also take -*ing*:

- *Give up*: Are you gonna *give up smoking*?
- *Keep on*: She *kept on interrupting* me while I was speaking.
- *Go on*: *Go on studying*, the exam will be next month.

When we are talking about finished actions, we can also use the verb *to have*:

- The resident *admitted forgetting* to change Mr. Smith's treatment.

or

- The resident *admitted having forgotten* to change Mr. Smith's treatment.

And, with some of these verbs (*admit, deny, regret* and *suggest*), you also can use a "that..." structure:

- The resident *admitted forgetting* to change Mr. Smith's treatment.

or

- The resident *admitted that he had forgotten* to change Mr. Smith's treatment.

Verb + Infinitive

When followed by another verb, these verbs are used with verb + infinitive structure:

- *Agree*: The patient *agreed to give up* smoking.
- *Refuse*: The patient *refused to give up* smoking.
- *Promise*: I *promised to give up* smoking.
- *Threaten*: Dr. Sommerset *threatened to close* the ward.
- *Offer*: The unions *offered to negotiate*.
- *Decide*: Dr. Knight's patients *decided to leave* the emergency room.

Other verbs that follow this structure are: *attempt, manage, fail, plan, arrange, afford, forget, learn, dare, tend, appear, seem, pretend, need*, and *intend*.

There are two possible structures after these verbs: *want, ask, expect, help, would like* and *would prefer*:

- Verb + infinitive: I *asked to see* Dr. Knight, the surgeon who operated on my patient.
- Verb + object + infinitive: I *asked Dr. Knight to inform* me about my patient.

There is only one possible structure after the following verbs: *tell, order, remind, warn, force, invite, enable, teach, persuade, get*:

- Verb + object + infinitive: *Remind me to report* those radiographs tomorrow before 10 a.m.

There are two possible structures after the following verbs:

- *Advise*:
  - I *wouldn't advise staying* at that hospital.
  - I *wouldn't advise you to stay* at that hospital.
- *Allow*:
  - They *don't allow smoking* in the OT.
  - They *don't allow you to smoke* in the OT.
- *Permit*:
  - They *don't permit eating* in the reporting room.
  - They *don't permit you to eat* in the reporting room.

When you use *make* and *let*, you should use the structure: verb + base form (instead of verb + infinitive):

- Blood *makes me feel* dizzy (you can't say: blood *makes me to feel*...).
- Dr. Knight *wouldn't let me operate on* his patient.

After the following expressions and verbs you can use either *-ing* or the infinitive: *like, hate, love, can't stand* and *can't bear*:

- She *can't stand being* alone.
- She *can't stand to be* alone.

After the following verbs you can use *-ing* but not the infinitive: *dislike, enjoy* and *mind*:

- I *enjoy being* alone (not: I *enjoy to be alone*).

Would like, a polite way of saying *I want*, is followed by the infinitive:

- *Would you like to be* the chairman of the congenital heart disease session?

Begin, start and *continue* can be followed by either *-ing* or the infinitive:

- The patient *began to improve* after intubation.
- The patient *began improving* after intubation.

With some verbs, like *remember* and *try*, the use of -ing and infinitive after them have different meanings:

- *Remember*:
  - *I did not remember to place* the tip of the catheter at the IVC before starting the contrast injection (I forgot to place the catheter properly).
  - *I could remember (myself) placing* the tip of a catheter at the IVC that day (I can recall placing the catheter).

- *Try*:
  - The patient *tried to keep* her eyes open.
  - If your headache persists, *try taking* an aspirin.

Verb + Preposition + -*Ing*

If a verb comes after a preposition, that verb ends in *-ing*:

- Are you *interested in working* for our hospital?
- *What are the advantages of developing* new surgical techniques?
- *She's not very good at learning* languages

You can use *-ing* with *before* and *after*:

- Discharge Mr. Brown *before operating* on the aneurysm.
- What did you do *after finishing* your residence?

You can use *by* + *-ing* to explain how something happened:

- You can improve your medical English *by reading* scientific articles.

You can use *-ing* after *without*:

- Jim got to the hospital *without realizing* he had left his locker keys at home.

Be careful with *to* because it can either be a part of the infinitive or a preposition:

- I'm looking forward to see you again (this is NOT correct).
- I'm looking forward to seeing you again.
- I'm looking forward to the next European congress.

Review the following verb + preposition expressions:

- *succeed in* finding a job
- *feel like* going out tonight
- *think about* operating on that patient
- *dream of* being a doctor
- *disapprove of* smoking
- *look forward to* hearing from you
- *insist on* inviting me to chair the session
- *apologize for* keeping Dr. Ho waiting
- *accuse* (someone) *of* telling lies
- *suspected of* having AIDS
- *stop from* leaving the ward
- *thank* (someone) *for* being helpful
- *forgive* (someone) *for* not writing to me
- *warn* (someone) *against* carrying on smoking

The following are some examples of expressions + *-ing*:

- *I don't feel like* going out tonight.
- *It's no use* trying to persuade her.
- *There's no point in* waiting for him.
- *It's not worth* taking a taxi. The hospital is only a short walk from here.
- *It's worth* looking again at that radiograph.
- *I am having difficulty* finding an apartment.
- *I am having trouble* finding an apartment.

Articles

Countable and Uncountable Nouns

Countable Nouns

Countable nouns are things we can count. We can make them plural.

Before singular countable nouns you may use *a/an*:

* You will be attended to by *a* cardiologist.
* Dr. Vida is looking for *an* anesthetist.

Remember to use *a/an* for jobs:

* I'm *a* surgeon.

Before plural countable nouns you use *some* as a general rule:

* I've read *some* good articles on spleen lately.

Don't use *some* when you are talking about general things:

* Generally speaking, I like radiology books.

You have to use *some* when you mean some, but not all:

* *Some* doctors carry a stethoscope but most of them don't.

Uncountable Nouns

Uncountable nouns are things we cannot count. They have no plural.

You cannot use *a/an* before an uncountable noun; in this case you have to use *the, some, any, much, this, his,* etc... or leave the uncountable noun alone, without the article:

* The chairman gave me an advice (NOT correct).
* The chairman gave me *some* advice.

Many nouns can be used as countable or uncountable nouns. Usually there is a difference in their meaning:

* I had *many experiences* on my rotation at the Children's Hospital (countable).
* I need *experience* to become a good surgeon (uncountable).

Some nouns are uncountable in English but often countable in other languages: *advice, baggage, behavior, bread, chaos, furniture, information, luggage, news, permission, progress, scenery, traffic, travel, trouble,* and *weather.*

A/An and *The*

The speaker says *a/an* when it is the first time he talks about something, but once the listener knows what the speaker is talking about, he says *the:*

- This morning I did *an* echography and *a* chest plain film. *The* echography was completely normal.

We use *the* when it is clear which thing or person we mean:

- Can you turn off *the* light.
- Where is *the* cardiology ward, please?

As a general rule, we say:

- The police
- The bank
- The post office
- The fire department
- The doctor
- The hospital
- The dentist

We say: *the* sea, *the* sky, *the* ground, *the* city, and *the* country.

We don't use *the* with the names of meals:

- What did you have for lunch/breakfast/dinner?

But we use *a* when there is an adjective before a noun:

- Thank you. It was *a* delicious dinner.

We use *the* for musical instruments:

- Can you play *the* piano?

We use *the* with absolute adjectives (adjectives used as nouns). The meaning is always plural. For example:

- The rich
- The old
- The blind
- The sick

- The disabled
- The injured
- The poor
- The young
- The deaf
- The dead
- The unemployed
- The homeless

We use *the* with nationality words (note that nationality words always begin with a capital letter):

- *The* British, *the* Dutch, *the* Spanish.

We don't use *the* before a noun when we mean something in general:

- I love doctors (not the doctors).

With the words *school, college, prison, jail, church* we use *the* when we mean the buildings and leave the substantives alone otherwise. We say: *go to bed, go to work* and *go home*. We don't use *the* in these cases.

We use *the* with geographical names according to the following rules:

- Continents don't use *the*:
  – Our new resident comes from Asia.

- Countries/states don't use *the*:
  – The patient that suffered a car accident came from Sweden.
  (except for country names that include words such as Republic, Kingdom, States...; e.g., the United States of America, the United Kingdom, and The Netherlands).

- As a general rule, cities don't use *the*:
  – The next Dermatology congress will be held in Madrid.

- Islands don't use *the* with individual islands but do use it with groups:
  – Dr. Holmes comes from Sicily and her husband from the Canary Islands.

- Lakes don't use *the*; oceans, seas, rivers and canals do use it.
  – Lake Windermere is beautiful.
  – *The* Panama canal links *the* Atlantic ocean to *the* Pacific ocean.

We use *the* with streets, buildings, airports, universities, etc, according to the following rules:

- Streets, roads, avenues, boulevards and squares don't use *the*:
  – The hospital is sited at 15th. Avenue.

- Airports don't use *the*:
  - The plane arrived at JFK airport

- We use *the* before publicly recognized buildings: *the* White House, *the* Empire State Building, *the* Louvre museum, *the* Prado museum.

- We use *the* before names with of: *the* Tower of London, *the* Great Wall of China.

- Universities don't use *the*: I studied at Harvard.

Word Order

The order of adjectives is discussed in the section Adjectives under the heading Adjective Order

The *verb* and the *object* of the verb normally go together:

- I studied medicine because I like *helping people* very much (not I like very much helping people).

We usually say the place before the time:

- She has been practicing interventional radiology in London since April.

We put some adverbs in the middle of the sentence:

- If the verb is one word we put the adverb before the verb:
  - I treated the patient and *also spoke* to his family.

- We put the adverb after *to be*:
  - You are *always* on time.

- We put the adverb after the first part of a compound verb:
  - Are you *definitely* attending the course?

- In negative sentences we put *probably* before the negative:
  - I *probably* won't see you at the congress.

- We also use *all* and *both* in these positions:
  - Jack and Tom have *both* applied for the job.
  - We *all* felt sick after the meal.

Relative Clauses

A clause is a part of a sentence. A relative clause tells us which person or thing (or what kind of person or thing) the speaker means.

A relative clause (e.g. *who is on call?*) begins with a relative pronoun (e.g. *who, that, which, whose*).

A relative clause comes after a noun phrase (e.g. the doctor, the nurse).

Most relative clauses are defining clauses and some of them are non-defining clauses.

Defining Clauses

The book on interventional radiology (that) you lent me is very interesting:

- The relative clause is essential to the meaning of the sentence.
- Commas are not used to separate the relative clause from the rest of the sentence.
- *That* is often used instead of who or which, especially in speech.
- If the relative pronoun is the object (direct object) of the clause, it can be omitted.
- If the relative pronoun is the subject of the clause, it cannot be omitted.

Non-Defining Clauses

The first cardiac transplant in the world, which took place in South Africa, was a complete success:

- The relative clause is not essential to the meaning of the sentence; it gives us additional information.
- Commas are usually used to separate the relative clause from the rest of the sentence.
- *That* cannot be used instead of who or which.
- The relative pronoun cannot be omitted.

Relative Pronouns

Relative pronouns are used for people and for things:

- For people:
  - Subject: *who, that*
  - Object: *who, that, whom*
  - Possessive: *whose*

- For things:
  - Subject: *which, that*
  - Object: *which, that*
  - Possessive: *whose*

Who is used only for people. It can be the subject or the object of a relative clause:

- The patient *who* was admitted in a shock situation is getting better.

Which is used only for things. Like *who*, it can be the subject or object of a relative clause:

- The materials *which* are used for embolization are very expensive.

That is often used instead of *who* or *which*, especially in speech.

Whom is used only for people. It is grammatically correct as the object of a relative clause, but it is very formal and is not often used in spoken English. We can use *whom* instead of *who* when *who* is the object of the relative clause or when there is a preposition after the verb of the relative clause:

- The resident *who* I am going to the congress with is very nice.
- The resident with *whom* I am going to the congress is a very nice and intelligent person.
- The patient *who* I saw in the ER yesterday has been diagnosed with Leriche's syndrome.
- The patient *whom* I saw in the ER yesterday has been diagnosed with Leriche's syndrome.

Whose is the possessive relative pronoun. It can be used for people and things. We cannot omit whose:

- Nurses *whose* wages are low should be paid more.

We can leave out *who, which* or *that*:

1. When it is the object of a relative clause.
   - The article on the spleen that you wrote is great.
   - The article on the spleen you wrote is great.
2. When there is a preposition. Remember that, in a relative clause, we usually put a preposition in the same place as in the main clause (after the verb):
   - The congress that we are going to next week is very expensive.
   - The congress we are going to next week is very expensive.

Prepositions in Relative Clauses

We can use a preposition in a relative clause with *who, which, that* or without a pronoun.

In relative clauses we put a preposition in the same place as in a main clause (after the verb). We don't usually put it before the relative pronoun. This is the normal order in informal spoken English:

- This is a problem *which* we can do very little about.
- The nurse (*who*) I spoke to earlier isn't here now.

In more formal or written English we can put a preposition at the beginning of a relative clause. But if we put a preposition at the beginning, we can only use *which* or *whom*. We cannot use the pronouns *that* or *who* after a preposition:

- This is a problem *about which* we can do very little.
- The nurse *to whom* I spoke earlier isn't here now.

Relative Clauses Without a Pronoun (Special Cases)

Infinitive Introducing a Clause

We can use the infinitive instead of a relative pronoun and a verb after:

1. The first, the second ... and the next
2. The only
3. Superlatives

For example:

- Roentgen was the first man *to use* X-rays.
- Joe was the only one *to discover* the diagnosis.

-Ing and -Ed Forms Introducing a Clause

We can use an *-ing* form instead of a relative pronoun and an active verb:

- Residents *wanting* to train abroad should have a good level of English.

We can use an *-ed* form instead of a relative pronoun and a passive verb:

- The man *injured* in the accident was taken to the hospital.

The *-ing* form or the *-ed* form can replace a verb in a present or past tense.

Why, When and Where

We can use *why*, *when* and *where* in a defining relative clause.

We can leave out *why* or *when*. We can also leave out *where*, but then we must use a preposition.

We can form non-defining relative clauses with *when* and *where*:

- The clinical history, *where* everything about a patient is written, is a very important document.

We cannot leave out *when* and *where* from a non-defining clause.

Adjectives

An adjective describes (tells us something about) a noun.

In English, adjectives come before nouns (old hospital) and have the same form in both the singular and the plural (new hospital, new hospitals) and in the masculine and in the feminine.

An adjective can be used with certain verbs such as *be, get, seem, appear, look* (meaning *seem*), *feel, sound, taste* ...:

- He has been *ill* since Friday.
- The patient was getting *worse*.
- The surgical intervention seemed *easy*, but it wasn't.
- The stools appear *black* when you are having iron orally.
- You look rather *tired*. Have you tested your RBC?
- She felt *sick*, so she went to see a doctor.
- Food in hospitals tastes *horrible*.

As you can see, in these examples there is no noun after the adjective.

Adjective Order

We have *fact adjectives* and *opinion adjectives*. Fact adjectives (large, new, white, ...) give us objective information about something (size, age, color, ...). Opinion adjectives (nice, beautiful, intelligent, ...) tell us what someone thinks of something.

In a sentence, opinion adjectives usually go before fact adjectives:

- An *intelligent* (opinion) *young* (fact) doctor visited me this morning.
- Dr. Spencer has a *nice* (opinion) *red* (fact) Porsche.

Sometimes there are two or more fact adjectives describing a noun, and generally we put them in the following order:

1. Size/length
2. Shape/width
3. Age
4. Color
5. Nationality
6. Material

For example:

- A tall young nurse
- A small round lesion
- A black latex leaded pair of gloves
- A large new white latex pair of gloves
- An old American patient
- A tall young Italian resident
- A small square old blue iron monitor

Regular Comparison of Adjectives

The form used for a comparison depends upon the number of syllables in the adjective:

Adjectives of one syllable: One-syllable adjectives (for example *fat, thin, tall*) are used with expressions of the form:

- less ... than (inferiority)
- as ... as (equality)
- -er ... than (superiority)

For example:

- Calls are *less hard than* a few years ago.
- Eating in the hospital is *as cheap as* eating at the Medical school.
- Nowadays people tend to be *fatter than* in the past.

Adjectives of two syllables: Two-syllable adjectives (for example *easy, dirty, clever*) are used with expressions of the form:

- less ... than (inferiority)
- as ... as (equality)
- -er/more ... than (superiority)

We prefer -er for adjectives ending in *y* (*easy, funny, pretty* ...) and other adjectives such as *quiet, simple, narrow, clever* .... For other two-syllable adjectives we use *more*.

For example:

- The clinical problem is *less simple than* you would think.
- My arm is *as painful as* it was yesterday.
- The board exam was *easier than* we expected.
- His illness was *more serious than* we first suspected.

Adjectives of three or more syllables: Adjectives of three or more syllables (for example *difficult, expensive, comfortable*) are used with expressions of the form:

- Less ... than (inferiority)
- As ... as (equality)
- More ... than (superiority)

For example:

- Studying medicine in Spain is *less expensive than* in the States.
- The small hospital was *as comfortable* as a hotel.
- Studying the case was *more interesting than* I had thought.

Before the comparative of adjectives you can use:

- A (little) bit
- A little
- Much
- A lot
- Far

For example:

- I am going to try something *much simpler* to solve the problem.
- The patient is *a little better* today.
- The little boy is *a little bit worse* today.

Sometimes it is possible to use two comparatives together (when we want to say that something is changing continuously):

- It is becoming *more and more* difficult to find a job in an academic hospital.

We also say *twice as ... as, three times as ... as*:

- Going to the European Congress of Paediatrics *is twice as expensive as* going to the French one.

The Superlative

The form used for a superlative depends upon the number of syllables in the adjective:

Adjectives of one syllable: One-syllable adjectives are used with expressions of the form:

- The ...-est
- The least

For example:

- Life expectancy in Spain is the second *highest* in the world.

Adjectives of two syllables: Two-syllable adjectives are used with expressions of the form:

- The ...-est/the most
- The least

For example:

- Hypertension is one of the *commonest* problems in clinical practice.
- Hypertension is one of the *most common* problems in clinical practice.

Adjectives of three or more syllables: Adjectives of three or more syllables are used with:

- The most
- The least

For example:

- Health and happiness are *the most important* things in a person's life.
- This is the *least difficult* case I have had in years.

Irregular Forms of Adjectives

- good   better   the best
- bad   worse   the worst
- far   farther/further   the farthest/furthest

For example:

- My headache is *worse* now than this morning in spite of having had two aspirins.

Comparatives with *The*

We use *the* + comparative to talk about a change in one thing which causes a change in something else:

- The higher our wages the better our standard of life.
- The more you practice the easier it gets.
- The higher the blood pressure the greater the risk of stroke.

As

Two things happening at the same time or over the same period of time:

- The resident listened carefully *as* Dr. Fraser explained to the patient the different treatment possibilities.
- I began to enjoy the residency more *as* I got used to being on call.

One thing happening during another:

- The patient died *as* the CT scan was being performed.
- I had to leave just *as* the clinical discussion was getting interesting.

Note that we use *as* only if two actions happen together. If one action follows another we don't use *as*, we use the particle *when*:

- *When* the injured person came to my ER, I decided to call the surgeon.

Meaning *because*:

- *As* I was feeling sick, I decided to go to the doctor.

Like and *As*

Like

Like is a preposition, so it can be followed by a noun, pronoun or *-ing* form.

It means *similar to* or *the same as*. We use it when we compare things:

- This quiet and comfortable hospital is *like* a good hotel.
- What does he do? He is a doctor, *like* me.

As

- *As* + subject + verb:
  - Don't change the treatment. Leave everything *as* it is.
  - He should have been treated *as* I showed you.

- Meaning *what*:
  - The resident did *as* he was told.
  - He made the diagnosis, *as* I expected.
  - *As* you know, we are sending an article to the European Journal of Radiology next week.
  - *As* I thought, the patient was under the influence of alcohol.

- *As* can also be a preposition, so it can be used with a noun, but it has a different meaning than like.

- *As* + noun is used to say what something really is or was (especially when we talk about someone's job or how we use something):
  - Before becoming a cardiologist I was working *as* a general practitioner in a small village.

- *As if*, *as though* are used to say how someone or something looks, sounds, feels, ... or to say how someone does something:
  - The doctor treated me as if I were his son.
  - John sounds as though he has got a cold.

- Expressions with *as*:
  - *Such as*
  - *As usual* (Dr. Mas was late *as usual*.)

So and Such

So and *such* make the meaning of the adjective stronger.

We use *so* with an adjective without a noun or with an adverb:

- The first year resident is *so clever*.
- The surgeon injected lidocaine *so carefully* that the patient did not notice it.

We use *such* with an adjective with a noun:

- She is *such a clever resident*.

Prepositions

At/On/In Time

- We use *at* with times:
  - *At* 7 o'clock
  - *At* midnight
  - *At* breakfast time

- We usually leave out *at* when we ask (*at*) *what time*:
  - *What time* are you operating this evening?

- We also use *at* in these expressions:
  - *At* night
  - *At* the moment
  - *At* the same time
  - *At* the beginning of
  - *At* the end of
  For example:
  - I don't like to be on call *at night*.
  - Dr. Knight is operating *at the moment*.

- We use *in* for longer periods of time:
  - *In* June
  - *In* summer
  - *In* 1977

- We also say *in the morning, in the afternoon, in the evening*:
  - I'll report all the MRI studies *in the morning*.

- We use *on* with days and dates:
  - *On* October 9th
  - *On* Monday
  - *On* Saturday mornings
  - *On* weekends (*At* weekends in British English)

- We do not use *at/in/on* before *last* and *next*:
  - I'll be on call *next* Saturday.
  - They bought a new CT *last* year.

- *In* + a period of time (i.e., a time in the future):
  - Our resident went to Boston. He'll be back *in* a year.

For, During and While

- We use *for* to say to how long something takes:
  - I've worked at this hospital *for* ten years.

- You cannot use *during* in this way:
  - It rained *for* five days (not *during* five days).

- We use *during* + noun to say when something happens (not how long):
  - The resident fell asleep *during* the operation.

- We use *while* + subject + verb:
  - The resident fell asleep *while* he was operating.

By and *Until*

- *By* + a time (i.e., not later than; you cannot use *until* with this meaning):
  - I mailed the article on carotid dissection today, so they should receive it *by* Tuesday.

- *Until* can be used to say how long a situation continues:
  - Let's wait *until* the patient gets better.

- When you are talking about the past, you can use *by the time*:
  - *By the time* they got to the hotel the congress had already started.

In/At/On

- We use *in* as in the following examples:
  - *In* a room
  - *In* a building
  - *In* a town/*in* a country (Dr. Vida works *in* Cordoba.)
  - *In* the water/ocean/river
  - *In* a row
  - *In* the hospital

- We use *at* as in the following examples:
  - *At* the bus stop
  - *At* the door/window
  - *At* the top/bottom
  - *At* the airport
  - *At* work
  - *At* sea
  - *At* an event (I saw Dr. Jules *at* the resident's party.)

- We use *on* as in the following examples:
  - *On* the ceiling
  - *On* the floor
  - *On* the wall
  - *On* a page
  - *On* your nose
  - *On* a farm

In or At?

- We say *in the corner of a room*, but *at the corner of a street*.

- We say *in* or *at* college/school. Use *at* when you are thinking of the college/school as a place or when you give the name of the college/school:
  - Thomas will be *in* college for three more years.
  - He studied medicine *at* Harvard Medical School.

- With buildings, you can use *in* or *at*.

- *Arrive*. We say:
  - *Arrive in* a country or town (Dr. Vida *arrived in* Boston yesterday.)
  - *Arrive at* other places (Dr. Vida *arrived at* the airport a few minutes ago.)
  - But: *arrive home* (Dr. Vida *arrived home* late after sending the article to AJR.)

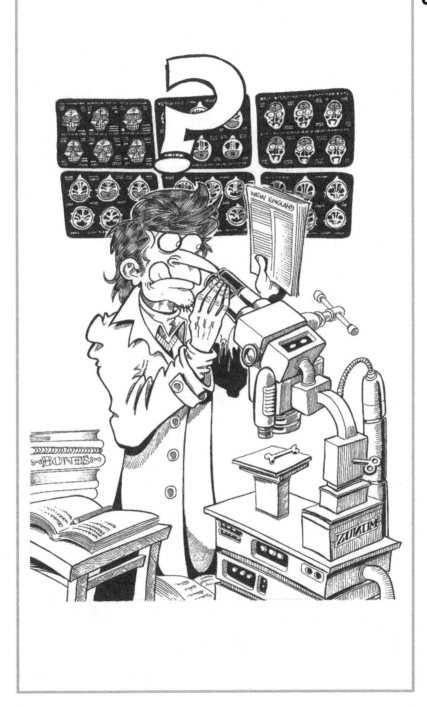

Unit III Scientific Literature

Writing an Article

This chapter is not intended to be a "Guide for Authors" such as those that you can find in any journal. Our main advice is: do not write the paper first in your own language and then translate it into English; instead, do it in English directly.

Preliminary Work

When you have a subject that you want to report, first of all you need to look up references. You can refer to the *Index Medicus* (http://www.ncbi.nlm.nih.gov/entrez/query.fcgi?db=PubMed) to search for articles. Once you have found them, read them thoroughly and underline those sentences or paragraphs that you think you might quote in your article.

Our advice is not to write the paper in your own language and then translate it into English; instead, do write in English directly. In order to do so, pick up, either out of these references, or out of the journal in which you want your work to be published, the article that you find closest to the type of study that you want to report.

Although you must follow the instructions of the journal to which you want to send the paper, here we will use a standard form that may be adequate for most of them. In each section, we will give you a few examples just to show how you can get them from other articles.

Article Header

Title

The title of the article should be concise but informative. Put a lot of thought into the title of your article.

Abstract

An abstract of 150–250 words (it depends on the journal) must be submitted with each manuscript. Remember that an abstract is a synopsis, *not* an introduction to the article.

The abstract should answer the question: "What should readers know after reading this article."

Most journals require that the abstract is divided into four paragraphs with the following headings.

Objective: To state the purposes of the study or investigation; the hypothesis being tested or the procedure being evaluated.

Notice that very often you may construct the sentence beginning with an infinitive tense:

* *To evaluate* the utility of curved planar reformations compared with standard transverse images in the assessment of pancreatic tumors.
* *To present* our experience of reconstruction of the chest wall after sternectomy for high-grade tumors.
* *To study* the diagnostic value of SPECT for multiple myeloma (MM).
* *To assess* ...
* *To compare* ...
* *To determine* ...
* *To perform* ...
* *To develop* ...
* *To demonstrate* ...
* *To investigate* ...
* *To ascertain* ...
* *To design* ...
* *To establish* ...

You can also begin with: "The aim/purpose of this study was to ...":

* *The aim of this study was to* adapt the Rheumatoid Arthritis Quality of Life (RAQoL) questionnaire for use in Turkey and to test its reliability and validity.
* *The purpose of this study was to* determine, on the basis of published reports, whether aspirin use during the first three months of pregnancy is associated with an increased risk of congenital malformations.
* *The goals of this study were to* define the natural history and growth pattern of hemangioblastomas of the central nervous system (CNS) that are associated with von Hippel-Lindau (VHL) disease and to correlate features of hemangioblastomas that are associated with the development of symptoms and the need for treatment.

- *The objective of this research was* two-fold: ...

You may give some background and then state what you have done.

- *This study was designed to ...*
- *We hypothesized that ...*
- *We compared ...*
- *We investigated ...*
- The relationship between liposarcoma and gene c-*myc* and p53 is not clear. There are also different reports on p53 mutation in liposarcoma. *This study was designed to* investigate the relationship between the expression of c-*myc* and p53 genes and liposarcomas.
- Although several early trials indicate treatment of restenosis with radiation therapy is safe and effective, the long-term impact of this new technology has been questioned. *The objective of this report is to* document angiographic and clinical outcome 3 years after treatment of restenotic stented coronary arteries with catheter-based ^{192}Ir.

Materials and Methods: Briefly state what was done and what materials were used, including the number of subjects. Also include the methods used to assess the data and to control bias.

- N *patients with ... were included.*
- N *patients known to have/suspected of having ...*
- *... was performed in N patients with ...*
- N *patients underwent ...*
- *Quantitative/Qualitative analyses were performed by ...*
- *Patients were followed clinically for ... months/years.*
- *We examined the effects of alcohol on blood pressure, heart rate, and forearm vascular resistance (FVR) during orthostatic stress achieved by stepwise increases in lower-body negative pressure (LBNP) in 14 healthy young volunteers.*

Results: Provide the findings of the study, including indicators of statistical significance. Include actual numbers, as well as percentages.

- *The clinical manifestations of the main kinds of intramedullary spinal cord tumors were not significantly different, but there were certain characteristic features in their neuroimage. The tumors of the grade 0 group (normal movement) were obviously smaller than those of other grade groups. The pre- and post-operative grades of motor disturbance showed a better, positive linear correlation.*

- *SPECT bone scan images of 44 patients were abnormal in the 46 patients with MM. The masculine rate was 95.6% ...*

Conclusion: Summarize in one or two sentences the conclusion(s) made on the basis of the findings. It should emphasize new and important aspects of the study or observations.

- *Improvement in stress blood flow and CFR is delayed compared with the lipid-lowering effect of fluvastatin, suggesting a slow recovery of the vasodilatory response to adenosine.*
- *MRI, particularly its enhancement, can differentiate an ependymoma from astrocytoma and hemangioblastoma in most cases. A satisfactory result can be achieved to enable resection of the tumor immediately by using minimally invasive, microsurgical techniques.*
- *Low p27(Kip1) expression is an independent adverse prognostic factor in patients with MM. The proposed risk score might be useful for risk-adapted treatment in the future.*
- *In conjunction with antitumor therapy, zoledronic acid should be considered for routine use to reduce skeletal complications in patients with advanced malignancies involving bone. In patients with hypercalcemia of malignancy, zoledronic acid is expected to become the treatment of choice.*
- *The study data demonstrate ...*

Keywords

Below the abstract you should provide, and identify as such, three to ten keywords or short phrases that will assist indexers in cross-indexing the article and may be published with the abstract. The terms used should be from the Medical Subject Headings list of the Index Medicus (http://www.nlm.nih.gov/mesh/meshhome.html).

Main Text

The text of observational and experimental articles is usually (but not necessarily) divided into sections with the headings *Introduction, Methods, Results,* and *Discussion.* Long articles may need subheadings within some sections (especially the Results and Discussion sections) to clarify their content. Other types of articles, such as Case Reports, Reviews, and Editorials, are likely to need other formats. You should consult individual journals for further guidance.

Avoid using abbreviations. When used, abbreviations should be spelled out the first time a term is given in the text, for example *magnetic resonance imaging (MRI).*

Introduction

The text should begin with an Introduction that conveys the nature and purpose of the work, and quotes the relevant literature. Give only strictly pertinent background information necessary for understanding why the topic is important and references that inform the reader as to why you undertook your study. Do not review the literature extensively. The final paragraph should clearly state the hypothesis or purpose of your study. Brevity and focus are important.

Materials and Methods

Details of clinical and technical procedures should follow the Introduction.

Describe your selection of the observational or experimental subjects (patients or laboratory animals, including controls) clearly. Identify the age, sex, and other important characteristics of the subjects. Because the relevance of such variables as age, sex, and ethnicity to the object of research is not always clear, authors should explicitly justify them when they are included in a study report. The guiding principle should be clarity about how and why a study was done in a particular way. For example, authors should explain why only subjects of certain ages were included or why women were excluded. You should avoid terms such as "race", which lack precise biological meaning, and use alternative concepts such as "ethnicity" or "ethnic group" instead. You should also specify carefully what the descriptors mean, and say exactly how the data were collected (for example, what terms were used in survey forms, whether the data were self-reported or assigned by others, etc.).

- *Our study population was selected from ...*
- *N patients underwent ...*
- *N consecutive patients ...*
- *N patients with proven ...*
- *Patients were followed clinically ...*
- *N patients with ... were examined before and during...*
- *N patients with known or suspected ... were prospectively enrolled in this study.*
- *More than N patients presenting with ... were examined with ... over a period of N months.*
- *N patients were prospectively enrolled between ... (date), and ... (date).*
- *N patients (N men, N women: age range, N–N years; mean, N±N years).*
- *In total, 141 children, aged 2 months to 4 years (mean 16 months), all with AEDS fulfilling the Hanifin–Rajka criteria, were included in the study.*

- *Patients undergoing elective coronary arteriography for evaluation of chest pain were considered eligible if angiography documented ...*

Identify the methods, instrumentation (trade names and manufacturer's name and location in parentheses), and procedures in sufficient detail to allow other workers to reproduce your study. Identify precisely all drugs and chemicals used, including generic name(s), dose(s), and route(s) of administration.

- *MR imaging was performed with a 1.5-T system (Vision; Siemens, Erlangen, Germany).*
- *The US-guided biopsy procedures were performed by using model RT 3000 equipment (GE Medical Systems, Milwaukee, Wis.) with either a 3.5- or a 5-MHz sector transducer combined with a needle guide or a 5-MHz linear-array transducer with a free-hand technique.*
- *Automatic high-speed core biopsy equipment (Biopty instrument and Biopty-Cut needles; Bard Urological, Covington, Ga.) was used.*
- *After baseline PET investigation, 40 mg of fluvastatin (Cranoc, Astra GmbH) was administered once daily.*
- *Dynamic PET measurements were performed with a whole-body scanner (CTI/ECAT 951R/31; Siemens/CTI). After a transmission scan for attenuation correction, 20 mCi of ^{13}N-labeled ammonia was administered as a bolus over 30 seconds by an infusion pump. The dynamic PET data acquisition consisted of varying frame durations (12×10 seconds, 6×30 seconds, and 3×300 seconds). For the stress study, adenosine was infused at a dose of $0.14 \, mg \cdot kg^{-1} \cdot min^{-1}$ over 5 minutes. ^{13}N-labeled ammonia was administered in a similar fashion as in the baseline study during the third minute of the adenosine infusion.*

It is essential that you state the manner by which studies were evaluated: independent readings, consensus readings, blinded or unblinded to other information, time sequencing between readings of several studies of the same patient or animal to eliminate recall bias, random ordering of studies. It should be clear as to the retrospective or prospective nature of your study.

- *Entry/inclusion criteria included ...*
- *These criteria had to be met: ...*
- *Patients with ... were not included.*
- *Further investigations, including ... and ..., were also performed.*
- *We prospectively studied N patients with ...*
- *The reviews were not blinded to the presence of ...*

- *The following patient inclusion criteria were used:* age between 16 and 50 years and closed epiphyses, ACL injury of one knee that required surgical replacement with a bone-to-patellar tendon-to-bone autograft, and signed informed consent with agreement to attend follow-up visits. *The following exclusion criteria were used*: additional ligament laxities with a grade higher than 2 (according to the European classification of frontal laxity) in the affected knee, ...
- Two skeletal radiologists (O.J., C.V.) *in consensus* studied the following parameters on successive MR images ...
- Both the interventional cardiologists and echocardiographers who performed the study and evaluated the results *were blinded to* drug administration.
- Histologic samples were evaluated *in a blinded manner* by one of the authors and an outside expert in rodent liver pathology.

Give references to established methods, including statistical methods that have been published but are not well known; describe new or substantially modified methods and give reasons for using these techniques, and evaluate their limitations. Identify precisely all drugs and chemicals used, including generic name(s), dose(s), and route(s) of administration. Do no use a drug's trade name unless it is directly relevant.

- *The imaging protocol included ...*
- *To assess objectively the severity of atopic dermatitis, all children were scored at each visit using the SCORAD method (10).*
- *The stereotactic device used for biopsy has been described elsewhere (12); it consists of a ...*
- *Gut permeability was measured in isolated intestinal segments as described previously (2).*

Statistics

Describe statistical methods with enough detail to enable a knowledgeable reader with access to the original data to verify the reported results. Put a general description of methods in the Methods section. When data are summarized in the Results section, specify the statistical methods used to analyze them:

- *A statistically significant difference was calculated with the Fisher exact test.*
- *The probability of ... was calculated by using the Kaplan-Meier method.*

- *To test for statistical significance, ...*
- *Statistical analyses were performed with ... and ... tests.*
- *The levels of significance are indicated by P values.*
- *Interobserver agreement was quantified by using k statistics.*
- *All P values of less than 0.05 were considered to indicate statistical significance.*
- *Univariate and multivariate Cox proportional hazards regression models were used.*
- *The χ^2-test was used for group comparison. Descriptive values of variables are expressed as means and percentages.*
- *We adjusted RRs for age (5-year categories) and used the Mantel extension test to test for linear trends. To adjust for other risk factors, we used multiple logistic regression.*

Give details about randomization:

- *They were selected consecutively by one physician between February 1999 and June 2000.*
- *This study was conducted prospectively during a period of 30 months from March 1998 to August 2000. We enrolled 29 consecutive patients who had ...*

Specify any general-use computer programs used:

- *All statistical analyses were performed with SAS software (SAS Institute, Cary, N.C.).*
- *The statistical analyses were performed by using a software package (SPSS for Windows, release 8.0; SPSS, Chicago, Ill.).*

Results

Present your results in logical sequence in the text, along with tables, and illustrations. Do not repeat in the text all the data in the tables or illustrations; emphasize or summarize only important observations. Avoid nontechnical uses of technical terms in statistics, such as "random" (which implies a randomizing device), "normal", "significant", "correlations", and "sample". Define statistical terms, abbreviations, and most symbols:

- *Statistically significant differences were shown for both X and X.*
- *Significant correlation was found between X and X.*
- *Results are expressed as means ±SD.*

- *All the abnormalities in our patient population were identified on the prospective clinical interpretation.*
- *The abnormalities were correctly characterized in 14 patients and incorrectly in ...*
- *The preoperative and operative characteristics of these patients are listed in Table 1.*
- *The results of the US-guided core-needle pleural biopsies are shown in Table 1.*
- *The clinical findings are summarized in Table 1.*

Report any complication:

- *Two minor complications were encountered. After the second procedure, one patient had a slight hemoptysis that did not require treatment, and one patient had local chest pain for about 1 hour after a puncture in the supraclavicular region. Pneumothorax was never encountered.*
- *Among the 11,101 patients, there were 373 in-hospital deaths (3.4%), 204 intraoperative/postoperative CVAs (1.8%), 353 patients with postoperative bleeding events (3.2%), and 142 patients with sternal wound infections (1.3%).*

Give numbers of observations. Report losses to observation (such as dropouts from a clinical trial):

- *The final study cohort consisted of ...*
- *Of the 961 patients included in this study, 69 patients were reported to have died (including 3 deaths identified through the NDI), and 789 patients were interviewed (Figure 1). For 81 surviving patients, information was obtained from another source. Twenty-two patients (2.3%) could not be contacted and were not included in the analyses because information on nonfatal events was not available.*

Discussion

Within this section, use ample subheadings. Emphasize the new and important aspects of the study and the conclusions that follow from them. Do not repeat in detail data or other material given in the Introduction or the Results sections. Include in the Discussion section the implications of the findings and their limitations, including implications for future research. Relate the observations to other relevant studies.

Link the conclusions with the goals of the study, but avoid unqualified statements and conclusions not completely supported by the data. In particular, avoid making statements on economic benefits and costs unless the report includes economic data and analyses. Avoid claiming priority and alluding to work that has not been completed. State new hypotheses when warranted, but clearly label them as such. Recommendations, when appropriate, may be included.

- *In conclusion, ...*
- *In summary, ...*
- *This study demonstrates that ...*
- *This study found that ...*
- *This study highlights ...*
- *Another finding of our study is ...*
- *One limitation of our study was ...*
- *Other methodological limitations of this study ...*
- *Our results support ...*
- *Further research is needed to understand ...*
- *However, the limited case number warrants a more comprehensive study to confirm these findings and to assess the comparative predictive value of relative lung volume versus LHR.*
- *Some follow-up is probably appropriate for these patients.*
- *Further research is needed when endoluminal surface coil technology is available.*

Acknowledgments

List all contributors who do not meet the criteria for authorship, such as a person who provided purely technical help, writing assistance, or a department chair who provided only general support. Financial and material support should also be acknowledged.

People who have contributed materially to the paper but whose contributions do not justify authorship may be listed under a heading such as "clinical investigators" or "participating investigators," and their function or contribution should be described: for example, "served as scientific advisors," "critically reviewed the study proposal," "collected data," or "provided and cared for study patients."

Because readers may infer their endorsement of the data and conclusions, everybody must have given written permission to be acknowledged.

- *The authors express their gratitude to ... for their excellent technical support.*
- *The authors thank Wei J. Chen, MD, ScD, Institute of Epidemiology, College of Public Health, National Taiwan University, Taipei, for the analysis of the statistics and his help in the evaluation of the data.*

The authors also thank Pan C. Yang, MD, PhD, Department *of Internal Medicine, and Keh S. Tsai, MD, PhD, Department of Laboratory Medicine, National Taiwan University, Medical College and Hospital, Taipei, for the inspiration and discussion of the research idea of this study. We also thank Ling C. Shen for her assistance in preparing the manuscript.*

References

References should be numbered consecutively in the order in which they are first mentioned in the text. Identify references in text, tables, and legends by Arabic numerals in parentheses (some journals require superscript Arabic numbers). References cited only in tables or figure legends should be numbered in accordance with the sequence established by the first citation in the text of the particular table or figure.

- *Clinically, resting thallium 201 (^{201}Tl) single photon emission computed tomography (SPECT) has been widely used to evaluate myocardial viability in patients with chronic coronary arterial disease and acute myocardial infarction (8–16).*
- *In addition, we have documented a number of other parameters previously shown to exhibit diurnal variation, including an assessment of sympathetic activity, as well as inflammatory markers recently shown to relate to endothelial function.*[14]

Use the style of the examples below, which are based on the formats used by the NLM in *Index Medicus.* The titles of journals should be abbreviated according to the style used in *Index Medicus.* Consult the *List of Journals Indexed in Index Medicus*, published annually as a separate publication by the library and as a list in the January issue of *Index Medicus.* The list can also be obtained through the library's website (http://www.nlm.nih.gov).

Avoid using abstracts as references. References to papers accepted but not yet published should be designated as "in press" or "forthcoming"; authors should obtain written permission to cite such papers as well as verification that they have been accepted for publication. Information from manuscripts submitted but not accepted should be cited in the text as "unpublished observations" with written permission from the source.

Avoid citing a "personal communication" unless it provides essential information not available from a public source, in which case the name of the person and date of communication should be cited in parentheses in the text. For scientific articles, authors should obtain written permission and confirmation of accuracy from the source of a personal communication.

The references must be verified by the author(s) against the original documents.

The Uniform Requirements style (the Vancouver style) is based largely on an ANSI standard style adapted by the NLM for its databases. Notes have been added where Vancouver style differs from the style now used by NLM.

Articles in Journals

Standard Journal Article

List the first six authors followed by et al. (Note: NLM now lists up through 25 authors; if there are more than 25 authors, NLM lists the first 24, then the last author, then et al.).

Vega KJ, Pina I, Krevsky B. Heart transplantation is associated with an increased risk for pancreatobiliary disease. Ann Intern Med 1996 Jun 1; 124 (11):980–3.

As an option, if a journal carries continuous pagination throughout a volume (as many medical journals do) the month and issue number may be omitted. (Note: For consistency, the option is used throughout the examples in Uniform Requirements. NLM does not use the option.)

Vega KJ, Pina I, Krevsky B. Heart transplantation is associated with an increased risk for pancreatobiliary disease. Ann Intern Med 1996; 124:980–3.

Organization as Author

The Cardiac Society of Australia and New Zealand. Clinical exercise stress testing. Safety and performance guidelines. Med J Aust 1996; 164: 282–4.

No Author Given

Cancer in South Africa [editorial]. S Afr Med J 1994; 84:15.

Article Not In English

(Note: NLM translates the title to English, encloses the translation in square brackets, and adds an abbreviated language designator.)

Galandi D, Allgaier HP. [Diet therapy in chronic inflammatory bowel disease: results from meta-analysis and randomized controlled trials] Schweiz Rundsch Med Prax. 2002 Nov 20; 91(47):2041–9. Review. German.

Volume with Supplement

Shen HM, Zhang QF. Risk assessment of nickel carcinogenicity and occupational lung cancer. Environ Health Perspect 1994; 102 Suppl 1:275–82.

Issue with Supplement

Payne DK, Sullivan MD, Massie MJ. Women's psychological reactions to breast cancer. Semin Oncol 1996; 23(1 Suppl 2):89–97.

Volume with Part

Ozben T, Nacitarhan S, Tuncer N. Plasma and urine sialic acid in non-insulin dependent diabetes mellitus. Ann Clin Biochem 1995; 32(Pt 3):303–6.

Issue with Part

Poole GH, Mills SM. One hundred consecutive cases of flap lacerations of the leg in ageing patients. N Z Med J 1994; 107(986 Pt 1):377–8.

Issue with No Volume

Turan I, Wredmark T, Fellander-Tsai L. Arthroscopic ankle arthrodesis in rheumatoid arthritis. Clin Orthop 1995; (320):110–4.

No Issue or Volume

Browell DA, Lennard TW. Immunologic status of the cancer patient and the effects of blood transfusion on antitumor responses. Curr Opin Gen Surg 1993:325–33.

Pages in Roman Numerals

Fisher GA, Sikic BI. Drug resistance in clinical oncology and hematology. Introduction. Hematol Oncol Clin North Am 1995 Apr; 9(2):xi–xii.

Type of Article Indicated as Needed

Enzensberger W, Fischer PA. Metronome in Parkinson's disease [letter]. Lancet 1996; 347:1337.
Clement J, De Bock R. Hematological complications of hantavirus nephropathy (HVN) [abstract]. Kidney Int 1992; 42:1285.

Article Containing Retraction

Garey CE, Schwarzman AL, Rise ML, Seyfried TN. Ceruloplasmin gene defect associated with epilepsy in EL mice [retraction of Garey CE, Schwarzman AL, Rise ML, Seyfried TN. In: Nat Genet 1994; 6:426–31]. Nat Genet 1995; 11:104.

Article Retracted

Liou GI, Wang M, Matragoon S. Precocious IRBP gene expression during mouse development [retracted in Invest Ophthalmol Vis Sci 1994; 35:3127]. Invest Ophthalmol Vis Sci 1994; 35:1083–8.

Article with Published Erratum

Hamlin JA, Kahn AM. Herniography in symptomatic patients following inguinal hernia repair [published erratum appears in West J Med 1995; 162:278]. West J Med 1995; 162:28–31.

Books and Other Monographs

Personal Author(s)

Ringsven MK, Bond D. Gerontology and leadership skills for nurses. 2nd ed. Albany (NY): Delmar Publishers; 1996.

(Note: Previous Vancouver style incorrectly had a comma rather than a semicolon between the publisher and the date.)

Editor(s), Compiler(s) as Author

Norman IJ, Redfern SJ, editors. Mental health care for elderly people. New York: Churchill Livingstone; 1996.

Organization as Author and Publisher

Institute of Medicine (US). Looking at the future of the Medicaid program. Washington: The Institute; 1992.

Chapter in a Book

Phillips SJ, Whisnant JP. Hypertension and stroke. In: Laragh JH, Brenner BM, editors. Hypertension: pathophysiology, diagnosis, and management. 2nd ed. New York: Raven Press; 1995. p. 465–78.

(Note: Previous Vancouver style had a colon rather than a p before pagination.)

Conference Proceedings

Kimura J, Shibasaki H, editors. Recent advances in clinical neurophysiology. Proceedings of the 10th International Congress of EMG and Clinical Neurophysiology; 1995 Oct 15–19; Kyoto, Japan. Amsterdam: Elsevier; 1996.

Conference Paper

Bengtsson S, Solheim BG. Enforcement of data protection, privacy and security in medical informatics. In: Lun KC, Degoulet P, Piemme TE, Rienhoff O, editors. MEDINFO 92. Proceedings of the 7th World Congress on Medical Informatics; 1992 Sep 6–10; Geneva, Switzerland. Amsterdam: North-Holland; 1992. p. 1561–5.

Scientific or Technical Report

Issued by funding/sponsoring agency: Smith P, Golladay K. Payment for durable medical equipment billed during skilled nursing facility stays. Final report. Dallas (TX): Dept. of Health and Human Services (US), Office of Evaluation and Inspections; 1994 Oct. Report No.: HHSIGOEI69200860. Issued by performing agency: Field MJ, Tranquada RE, Feasley JC, editors. Health services research: work force and educational issues. Washington: National Academy Press; 1995. Contract No.: AHCPR282942008. Sponsored by the Agency for Health Care Policy and Research.

Dissertation

Kaplan SJ. Post-hospital home health care: the elderly's access and utilization [dissertation]. St. Louis (MO): Washington Univ.; 1995.

Patent

Larsen CE, Trip R, Johnson CR, inventors; Novoste Corporation, assignee. Methods for procedures related to the electrophysiology of the heart. US patent 5,529,067. 1995 Jun 25.

Other Published Material

Newspaper Article

Lee G. Hospitalizations tied to ozone pollution: study estimates 50,000 admissions annually. The Washington Post 1996 Jun 21; Sect. A:3 (col. 5).

Audiovisual Material

HIV+/AIDS: the facts and the future [videocassette]. St. Louis (MO): Mosby Year-Book; 1995.

Dictionary and Similar References

Stedman's medical dictionary. 26th ed. Baltimore: Williams & Wilkins; 1995. Apraxia; p. 119–20.

Unpublished Material

In Press
(Note: NLM prefers "forthcoming" because not all items will be printed.)

Leshner AI. Molecular mechanisms of cocaine addiction. N Engl J Med. In press 1996.

Electronic Material

Journal Article in Electronic Format

Morse SS. Factors in the emergence of infectious diseases. Emerg Infect Dis [serial online] 1995 Jan-Mar [cited 1996 Jun 5]; 1(1):[24 screens]. Available from: URL: http://www.cdc.gov/ncidod/EID/eid.htm.

Monograph in Electronic Format

CDI, clinical dermatology illustrated [monograph on CD-ROM]. Reeves JRT, Maibach H. CMEA Multimedia Group, producers. 2nd ed. Version 2.0. San Diego: CMEA; 1995.

Computer File

Hemodynamics III: the ups and downs of hemodynamics [computer program]. Version 2.2. Orlando (FL): Computerized Educational Systems; 1993.

Tables

All tabulated data identified as tables should be given a table number and a descriptive caption. Take care that each table is cited in numerical sequence in the text.

The presentation of data and information given in the table headings should not duplicate information already given in the text. Explain in footnotes all non-standard abbreviations used in the table.

If you need to use any table or figure from another journal, make sure you ask for permission and put a note such as:

Adapted, with permission, from reference 5.

Figures

Figures should be numbered consecutively according to the order in which they are first cited in the text. Follow the "pattern" of similar illustrations of your references.

- *Figure 1. Nonenhanced CT scan shows ...*

- *Figure 2. Contrast-enhanced CT scan obtained at the level of ...*

- *Figure 3. Selective renal arteriogram shows ...*

- *Figure 4. Photograph of the fresh cut specimen shows ...*

- *Figure 5. Photomicrograph (original magnification, ×10; hematoxylin-eosin stain) of ...*

- *Figure 6. Coronal contrast-enhanced T1-weighted MR image of ...*

- *Figure 7. Typical metastatic compression fracture in a 65-year-old man. (a) Sagittal T1-weighted MR image (400/11) shows ...*

- *Figure 6. Nasal-type extranodal NK/T-cell lymphoma involving the nasal cavity in a 42-year-old woman. Photomicrograph (original magnification, ×400; hematoxylin-eosin [H-E] stain) of a nasal mucosal biopsy specimen shows intense infiltration of atypical lymphoid cells into the vascular intima and subintima (arrow). This is a typical appearance of angiocentric invasion in which the vascular lumen (V) is nearly obstructed.*
- *Figure 7. AFX with distortion of histopathologic architecture as a consequence of intratumoral hemorrhage.*
- *Figure 8. CT images obtained in a 75-year-old man with gross hematuria. (a) MIP image obtained during the compression-release excretory phase demonstrates a nonobstructing calculus (arrow) in the distal portion of the right ureter.*

Final Tips

Before you submit your article for publication check its spelling, and go over your article for words you might have omitted or typed twice, as well as words you may have misused such as using "there" instead of "their." Do not send an article with spelling or dosage errors or other medical inaccuracies. And don't expect the spell-check function on your computer to catch all your spelling mistakes.

Be accurate. Check and double-check your facts and reference citations. Even after you feel the article is finished leave it for a day or two and then go back to it. The changes you make to your article after seeing it in a new light will often be the difference between a good article and a great article.

Once you believe everything is correct, give the draft to your English teacher for a final informal editing. Do not send your first (or even second) draft to the publisher!

Do not forget to read and follow carefully the specific "Instructions for authors" of the journal in which you want your work to be published.

Letters

Submission

The following is an example of a covering letter to accompany an article submitted to a journal:

Your address

Addressee's name

Destination address

Date (in the form 2 January 2003)

Dear Dr. ...:

Please find enclosed N copies of our manuscript entitled "..." (authors ..., ..., ...), which we hereby submit for publication in... [name of journal]. Also enclosed is a diskette with a copy of the text file in Microsoft Word for Windows (version N).

I look forward to hearing from you.

Yours sincerely,

Dr. Vida

Resubmission

The following is an example of a covering letter to accompany an article on resubmission:

Your address

Addressee's name

Destination address

Date (in the form 10 February 2003)

Dear Dr....:

In reply to your letter of 3 February 2003, please find enclosed N copies of the new version of our manuscript ref. XXXX entitled "..." (authors ..., ..., ...), which has been carefully revised in light of your comments and those of the referees, as detailed on the attached sheets.

We hope that this revised version will now be judged ready for publication in ... [name of journal], and look forward to hearing from you.

Yours sincerely,

Dr. Vida

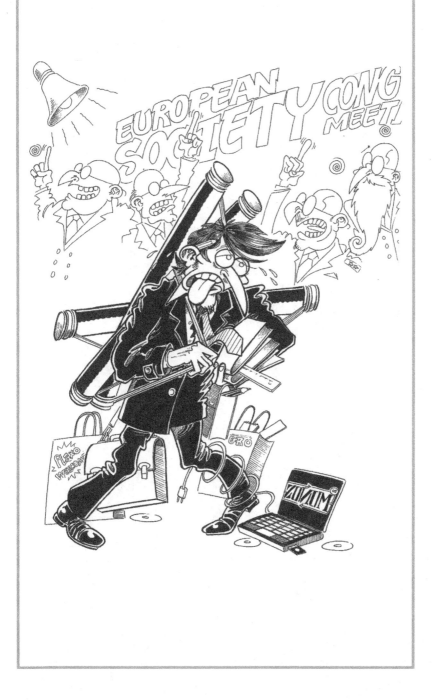

Unit IV Talks and Courses

Introduction

In the following pages we take a look inside international medical meetings. We recommend upper-intermediate English speakers to quickly go over them and intermediate English speakers to review this section thoroughly in order to become familiar with the jargon of international congresses.

Course Example

We take as an example the 5th European Congress of Endocrinology which will be held in the city of Turin (Northern Italy) from 9 to 13 June 2001.

Program Planning

We first discuss the scientific program as set out in Table 1. The elements of the program in Table 1 are explained more fully as follows:

- *Satellite symposia:* Scientific events sponsored by pharmaceutical firms where new drugs, techniques or devices are presented to the medical community.
- *Plenary lecture:* This event takes place usually both at the beginning and at the end of the day gathering all participants around an outstanding member of the medical community.
- *Symposia:* Conferences divided into three to five sections, of 30 to 45 minutes each and conducted by different experts. They are focused on different aspects (pathophysiology, diagnosis, treatment strategies, controversial facts, etc.) of a given matter.

Table 1. 5th European Congress of Endocrinology plan

	Saturday, June 9	Sunday, June 10	Monday, June 11	Tuesday, June 12	Wednesday, June 13
Morning	Satellite symposia	Plenary lecture Symposia Free communications	Plenary lecture Symposia Free communications	Plenary lecture Symposia Free communications	Plenary lecture Symposia Free communications
Afternoon	Opening ceremony Plenary lecture	Posters Meet the expert Symposia Free communications Plenary lecture	Posters Meet the expert Symposia Free communications Plenary lecture	Posters Meet the expert Symposia Free communications Plenary lecture	Closing ceremony
Evening	Welcome cocktail	EFES General Assembly	EFES General Assembly		
Late evening	Concert		Social dinner		

- *Free communications:* In this section, the Scientific Committee selects, from all the abstracts submitted, the most outstanding basic and clinical research works, and invites the authors to perform a presentation of their methods and conclusions (usually not longer than 10 to 15 minutes). A round of questions and/or comments is usually permitted.
- *Meet the expert:* Scientific authorities are invited by the Organizing Committee to present their recent investigations or clinical work-up. Participation by the public is encouraged.

Registration Form

The registration form takes the following form:
* Please, fill out and return the registration form to the organizing secretariat by fax or mail with the appropriate payment made payable to the International Congress Centre, Via Cervino, 60, 10155 Torino, Italy.

Please complete in BLOCK CAPITALS (i.e., upper case letters):
Surname: . . . .
Given name: . . . .
Title/post (e.g., Consultant, Attending,
Professor, Chairman, Radiographer): . . . .
Department: . . . .
Institution (e.g., Hospital, Medical Center): . . . .
Address: . . . .
Post code: . . . .
City: . . . .
Country: . . . .
Telephone: . . . .
Fax: . . . .
E-mail: . . . .

Registration

Full Registration

Full registration includes:
* Access to all congress sessions, to satellite symposia and commercial exhibition
* Document case with program
* Abstract book and abstract in CD-ROM
* Welcome reception
* Coffee breaks
* Lunches
* Shuttle bus service to congress venue
* Coupons for discount price dinners are available.
Fees per person (including 20% VAT):
* Early registration € 400.00
* Late registration € 475.00

Student Registration

Student registration includes:
- Access to all congress sessions and commercial exhibition
- Document case with program
- Abstract book and abstract in CD-ROM
- Welcome reception
- Coffee breaks
- Lunches
- Shuttle bus service to congress venue
- Coupons for discount price dinners.

Fees per person (including 20% VAT):
- Early registration € 275.00
- Late registration € 350.00

Special economic package

The special economic package is for 500 persons only and includes:
- Access to all congress sessions, to satellite symposia and commercial exhibition
- Document case with program
- Abstract book and abstract in CD-ROM
- Welcome reception
- Coffee breaks
- Lunches
- Hotel accommodation (4 days in double room)
- Shuttle bus service to congress venue

Fee per person (including 20% VAT):
- Anytime registration € 520.00

Accompanying Person Registration

Accompanying person registration includes:
- Access to all congress sessions and commercial exhibition
- Document case with program
- Welcome reception
- Coffee breaks
- Lunches
- Shuttle bus service to congress venue
- Coupons for discount price dinners

Fee per person (including 20% VAT):
- Anytime registration € 250.00

Social dinner, 11 June 2001

Fee per person (including 20% VAT):
* Anytime registration € 100.00

Methods of Payment

Bank Transfer

Bank transfer to:
* International Congress Centre. Banca di Sicilia Agenzia 2. Corso Francia, 25, Torino (Italy). Account # 410/612661.

Check

International bank check or personal check not transferable, made payable to: International Congress Centre.
* Check number: ....
* Bank: ....

Credit Card

Please provide the following information:
* Visa/Eurocard/Mastercard/American Express
* Card number: ....
* Expiry date: ....
* Card holder's name: ....
* Card holder's date of birth: ....
* Place of residence: ....
* Signature: ....

General Information

The Congress

Language
The official language of the congress will be English.

Dress Code
Formal dress is required for the Opening Ceremony and for the Social Dinner. Casual wear is acceptable for all other events and occasions.

Commercial Exhibition
Participants will have the opportunity to visit representatives from pharmaceutical, diagnostic and equipment companies, and publishers at their stands to discuss new developments and receive up-to-date product information.

Local Information

Passport and Visa

A valid passport or identity card is enough to enter Italy from most countries (EU, USA, Canada, Australia, etc) while a visa is required for citizens of other countries (People's Republic of China, Russia, India, etc). For further information contact the nearest Italian embassy.

How to Reach Turin
Turin lies on the main Italian motorway network (A4, A5, A6, A21) with good connections to other European systems: Milan (1.5 h), Genoa (2 h), Nice (3 h), Paris (8 h). By air, Turin is served by the City of Turin Caselle Airport, located 16 km from the center. Flights are available on European and domestic routes with daily connections to Paris, London, Amsterdam, Brussels, Zurich, Barcelona, Madrid, Lisbon, Rennes, Frankfurt, Munich, Stuttgart, Düsseldorf, and frequent flights to Rome.

Hence, Turin can be reached from most European capitals at rates comparable to mid-range distances. The airline companies operating these services include: Alitalia, Aerolineas Argentinas, Air France, Air Malta, British Airways, British Caledonian Airways, Iberia, KLM, Lufthansa, Sabena, SAS, Swissair, Thai-Air, TWA, Varig, and World Jet. Turin is connected by rail to the rest of Europe through France and Germany. Good connections include Intercity services to Rome, Milan, Venice, and Trieste, and the TGV direct to Paris. Located in the city center, the main railway station, *Porta Nuova*, is within walking distance of many hotels.

Financial Matters

The common European currency is the Euro.

Banks in Italy are open from 08.30 to 13.00 and from 14.50 to 16.00 Monday to Friday. Banks are closed on Saturday and Sunday. As is usual, money exchange facilities, ATMs/cashpoints and car rental outlets are available at the airport, in the city center, and at most hotels.

Weather

The weather in Turin in June is usually rather warm with occasional rain. The daytime temperatures normally range from 14 °C to 25 °C (55–77 °F).

Giving a Talk

International medical conferences are in a universe all of their own. In this universe, attendees and speakers come from many different countries with their own cultures and consequently their own habits in terms of behavior and public speaking. However, most speakers set aside, at least partially, their cultural identity to embrace the international medical conference style. This standardization is part of the globalization that we are all witnessing.

The most widely spoken language is not Chinese, English or Spanish anymore, but the new phenomenon of broken English. This language is the result of simplifying English to make it as neutral and understandable as possible, removing colloquial idioms, regional expressions or any other linguistic source of confusion.

In this new universe, health-care professionals find themselves having to make a conscious effort to adapt to these explicit and implicit rules. Some of them are discussed in the following sections.

Do's and Don'ts

Time is also a very cultural thing. This peculiarity should be taken into account. Eight o'clock in the morning might seem an early start in Latin America but a perfectly normal starting time in northern Europe and the US. Furthermore, the day is divided differently in various parts of the world ... and in our medical universe. Thus at an international conference the day is divided into:

- The morning: from the start time to 12:00
- The afternoon: from 12:01 to 17:00 or 18:00
- The evening: from 18:00 to midnight.

Do remember to follow these tips:

* Good morning: from starting time to 12:00.
* Good afternoon: from 12:01 onwards, even though our metabolism is far from feeling afternoon-ish and is begging us to say "good morning".
* Good evening: from 18:00 onwards. Note that if we have to give a presentation, make a speech or offer a toast at 22:00, we should never begin with "good night"; that should be reserved only for when we are going to bed.

When giving a presentation, there is always a time limit. I understand, and have actually experienced myself, how difficult it is to cram all we have to say about the topic which we have been researching over the last few years into a mere 20 minutes. In view of this time constraint, there are various alternatives ranging from speaking as fast as the tongue can rattle, to cutting it down to 5 minutes and spending the other 15 minutes vacantly gazing at the audience. American, British and Australian physicians are often extremely fluent speakers (we know, we know ... they are using their mother tongue). However, remember that showing and commenting on five slides a minute and speaking faster than can be registered on a digital recorder might not be the best way of conveying a message.

* *Don't* speak too fast or too slowly.
* *Do* summarize your presentation and rehearse to see how long you need for clear delivery.

Sometimes lecturers tend to give too much data and minor details in their presentations. Their introduction is often full of information that is of little relevance for the international audience (for example, the name, date and code of local, provincial, regional and national laws regulating health-care standards in his/her institution; or even the background information on the main researchers of a trial including their graduation year and shoe size ... or a full history of the 16th Century building where the hospital stands today and subsequent restorations it has undergone; etc). In these cases, by the time all these details have been given and the presentation has passed the introduction stage, time is up and the chairperson starts making desperate signs to the speaker.

* *Do* structure your presentation so that you convey a few clear messages instead of a huge amount of not-so-relevant information which nobody has a chance to take in.
* *Don't* read from a script, but instead try to explain a few basic ideas as clearly as possible. Many intermediate English-speaking doctors could not agree with this point because they can only feel some confidence if they read the presentation. Reading is the least-natural means of communicating experiences; we encourage you to present your paper without reading it. Although it will need much more intensive preparation, the delivery will be more fluid and – why not? – even brilliant. Many

foreign doctors resign themselves to delivering just acceptable talks and explicitly reject the possibility of making a presentation at the same level as in their own language. Do not reject the possibility of being as brilliant as you would be in your own language; the only difference consists in rehearsing. Thorough rehearsal can provide you with amazing results; do not give up beforehand.

Enjoy yourself. When giving the presentation relax; nobody knows more than you do about the specific subject that you are presenting. The only way to make people enjoy your presentation is by enjoying it yourself. You only have to communicate, not to perform; being a good researcher or a competent clinician is not the same thing as being a stand-up comedian or a model. This does not mean that we can afford to overlook our presentation skills, especially if you want most of your colleagues to still be awake at the end of your presentation!

- *Do* try to overcome stage fright and focus on communicating. There must be somebody out there interested in what you have to say ... either to praise it or to tear it to pieces, but that doesn't matter.
- *Do* avoid anything that would make you nervous when giving your presentation. One piece of advice is to remove all keys, coins or other metal objects from your pockets so that you are not tempted to rattle them around – a truly irritating noise that we have all learned to hate.

Humor ... what can we say about humor? We all know that humor is a very cultural thing, like timekeeping, ties, food preferences, etc. Almost all American speakers will start their presentation with a joke that most Europeans will not understand, not even the Irish or British. A British speaker will probably throw in the most sarcastic comment when you are least expecting it and in the same tone as if he or she were telling you about the mortality rate in his or her unit. A foreign (neither American nor British) doctor might just try to tell a long joke in English based on a play on words in his or her mother tongue which obviously doesn't work in English and possibly involves religion, football and/or sex (as a general rule avoid religious and sex jokes in public presentations).

- *Do* make sure that your jokes can be understood internationally. Creativity and humor are always appreciated in a lecture hall ... providing they are both appropriate and understood!

Chairing a Session

Chairing sessions at international meetings usually comes up when you have reached a certain level in your academic career. To reach this point many papers will have been submitted and many presentations will have been given, so the chances are your medical English level will be above that of the target audience of this manual.

Why, then, do we include a section on chairing a session?

We include it because contrary to what many of those who have never chaired a session in an international meeting may think, even an experienced chairperson might face difficult, even embarrassing situations.

For those who have never chaired a session, to be a chairman means, firstly, not having to prepare a presentation, and, secondly, the use of simple sentences such as "thank you, Dr. Vida, for your interesting presentation" or "the next speaker will be Dr. Jones who comes from …".

In our opinion, being a chairperson means much more than those who have never chaired them might think. To begin with, a chairperson must go over not one presentation but thoroughly study all the recently published material on the discussed subject. On top of that, a chairperson must review all the abstracts and must have prepared questions just in case the audience has no questions or comments.

We have divided this section into three subsections:

1. Usual chairperson's comments.
2. Should chairpersons ask questions?
3. What the chairperson should say when something is going wrong.

Usual Chairperson's Comments

Everybody who has attended an international meeting is aware of the usual sentences the chairperson uses to introduce the session. Certain key expressions will provide you with a sense of fluency without which chairing a session would be troublesome. The good news is that if you know the key sentences and use them appropriately, chairing a session is easy. The bad news is that if, on the contrary, you do not know these expressions, a theoretically simple task will become an embarrassing situation.

Introducing the Session

We suggest the following useful comments for introducing the session:

- Good morning ladies and gentlemen. My name is Dr. Vida and I want to welcome you all to this workshop on congenital heart disease. My co-chair is Dr. Vick who comes from King's College.
- Good afternoon. The session on cardiomyopathies is about to start. Please take a seat and disconnect your cellular phones and any other electrical devices which could interfere with the oral presentations. We will listen to ten 6-minute lectures with a 2-minute period for questions and comments after each of them, and afterwards, provided we are still on time, we will have a last round of questions and comments from the audience, speakers and panelists.

- Good morning. We will proceed with the session on fibroid embolization. As many papers have to be delivered I encourage the speakers to
  keep an eye on the time.

Introducing Speakers
We suggest the following useful comments for introducing speakers:

- Our first speaker is Dr. Vida from Reina Sofia Hospital in Cordoba, Spain,
  who will present the paper: "MR evaluation of focal splenic lesions".

The following speakers are introduced almost the same way with sentences
such as:

- Our next lecturer is Dr. Adams. Dr. Adams comes from Brigham and
  Women's Hospital. Harvard Medical School, and his presentation is en-
  titled "Diagnosis and treatment of hemangiopericytoma".
- Next is Dr. Shaw from Beth Israel Deaconess Hospital, presenting "Sur-
  gical treatment of insulinomas".
- Dr. Olsen from UCSF is the next and last speaker. His presentation is:
  "Metastatic disease. Pathways to the heart".

Once the speakers finish their presentation, the chairperson is supposed to
say something like:

- Thank you Dr. Vida for your excellent presentation. Any questions or
  comments?

The chairperson usually comments on presentations, although sometimes
they do not do it:

- Thank you Dr. Vida for your presentation. Are there any questions or
  comments from the audience?

There are some common adjectives (nice, elegant, outstanding, excellent,
interesting, clear, accurate ...) and formulas that are usually used to describe presentations. These are illustrated in the following comments:

- Thanks Dr. Shaw for your accurate presentation. Does the audience have
  any comments?
- Thank you very much for your clear presentation on this always controversial topic. I would like to ask a question. May I? (Although being the
  chairperson you are the one who gives permission, to ask the speaker is
  a usual formality.)
- I'd like to thank you for this excellent talk Dr. Olsen. Any questions?
- Thanks a lot for your talk Dr. Ho. I wonder if the audience has got any
  questions?

There is always a first time for everything, and if it is the first time you have been invited to chair a session, rehearse some of the sentences above and you will feel quite comfortable. Accept this piece of advice: only "rehearsed spontaneity" looks spontaneous if you are a beginner.

Adjourning
We suggest the following useful comments for adjourning the session:

- I think we all are a bit tired so we'll have a short break.
- The session is adjourned until 4 pm.
- We'll take a short break.
- We'll take a 30 minute break. Please fill out the evaluation forms.
- The session is adjourned until tomorrow morning. Enjoy your stay in San Francisco.

Finishing the Session
We suggest the following useful comments for finishing the session:

- I'd like to thank all the speakers and the audience for your interesting presentations and comments. (I'll) see you all at the congress dinner and awards ceremony.
- The session is over. I want to thank all the participants for their contribution. (I'll) see you tomorrow morning. Remember to take your attendance certificates if you have not taken them already.
- We should finish up over here. We'll resume at 10:50.

Should Chairpersons Ask Questions?

In our opinion, chairpersons are supposed to ask questions especially at the beginning of the session when the audience does not usually make any comments at all. Warming-up the session is one of the chairperson's duties and if nobody in the audience is in the mood to ask questions the chairperson must invite the audience to participate:

- Are there any questions?

Nobody raises their hand:

- Well, I have got two questions for Dr. Adams: Do you think MR is the imaging method of choice for the detection and characterization of focal splenic lesions? and second: What should be, in your opinion, the role of CT and ultrasound in this diagnostic algorithm?

Once the session has been warmed-up, the chairperson should only ask questions or add comments as a tool to manage the timing of the session, so that, if as usual, the session is behind schedule, the chairperson is not required to participate unless strictly necessary.

The chairperson does not have to demonstrate to the audience his or her knowledge on the discussed topics by asking too many questions or making comments. The chairperson's knowledge of the subject is not in doubt since without it he or she would not have been selected to chair.

What the Chairperson Should Say when Something is Going Wrong

Behind Schedule

Many lecturers, knowing beforehand they have a certain amount of time to deliver their presentations, try to talk a little bit more stealing time from the questions/comments time and from later speakers. Chairpersons should cut short this tendency at the very first chance:

- Dr. Berlusconi, your time is almost over. You have got 30 seconds to finish your presentation.
- Dr. Ho, you are running out of time.

If the speaker does not finish his presentation on time, the chairperson may say:

- Dr. Berlusconi, I'm sorry but your time is over. We must proceed to the next presentation. Any questions, comments?

After introducing the next speaker, sentences like the following ones will help you to handle the session:

- Dr. Goyen, please keep an eye on the time, we are behind schedule.
- We are far from being ahead of schedule, so I remind all speakers you have 6 minutes to deliver your presentations.

Ahead of Schedule

Although unusual, sometimes there is some extra time and this is a good chance to ask the panelists a general question about their experience at their respective institutions:

- As we are a little bit ahead of schedule, I encourage the panelists and the audience to make questions and comments.
- I have got a question for the panelists: What percentage of the total number of CMRs at your institution are performed on children?

Technical Problems
Computer Not Working

We suggest the following comments:

- I am afraid there is a technical problem with the computer. In the meantime I would like to make a comment about ...
- The computer is not working properly. While it is being fixed I encourage the panelists to make their always interesting comments.

Lights Gone Off
We suggest the following comments:

- The lights have gone off. We'll make a hopefully short stop until it is repaired.
- As you see, or better, do not see at all, the lights have gone off. The hotel staff have told us it is going to be a matter of minutes so do not go too far; we'll resume as soon as possible.

Sound Gone Off
We suggest the following comments:

- Dr. Hoffman, we cannot hear you. There must be a problem with your microphone.
- Would you try this other microphone?
- Would you please use the microphone, the rows at the back cannot hear you.

Lecturer Lacks Confidence
If the lecturer is speaking too quietly:

- Dr. Smith would you please speak up? The audience cannot hear you.
- Dr. Alvarez would you please speak up a bit? The people at the back cannot hear you.

If the lecturer is so nervous he/she cannot go on delivering the presentation:

- Dr. Olson, take your time. We can proceed to the next presentation, so whenever you feel OK and ready to deliver yours, it will be a pleasure to listen to it.

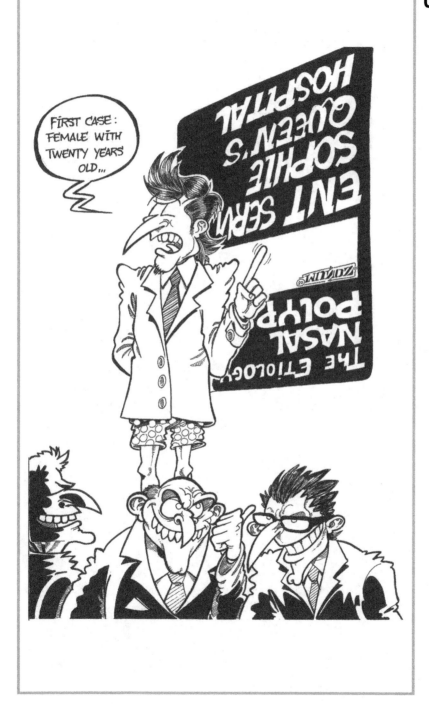

Unit V Some of the Most Frequent Mistakes Made by Doctors Speaking in English

What Can Go Wrong ... Nightmares That Don't Come True

What? A section on nightmares? As in bad dreams that make you wake up in the middle of the night? Or a section on things that could go wrong in life, i.e., buying a used car on the black market? Or both? Or neither?

We could just hear the reader mumbling these questions when scanning through the table of contents just as his/her finger hovers over this title. Yes, this is indeed a section only for the brave, only for those who have actually made it all the way here to this page, to face the jungle out there. The jungle being the challenge of *preparing and delivering a presentation in English when one is just a simple mortal.*

We have decided to write about this topic because we ourselves used to be the ones with nightmares. There were so many things that could go wrong when dealing with medical terminology in English, that the mathematical concept of infinity seemed ridiculously small.

In this section we try and share with you what we have found to be some of the great hurdles in medical English. There are many things that certainly *can* go wrong when one is asked to give a lecture in English. This is by no means an exhaustive account from a comprehensive risk assessment study. Rather it is just a way of passing on what we have learnt from our own experience in the fascinating world of international medical conferences.

As mentioned before in this book, many doctors did not have a lucky day when Mother Nature handed out predisposing factors for success at giving presentations in English. Firstly, they did not live in a country where English is part of day-to-day life. Secondly, they were never taught languages properly at school.

When preparing and actually delivering a presentation in English at an international medical conference, a series of basic issues should be taken into account. We have grouped them into three danger zones, in the hope that their classification will make them shrink or at least become less of a problem. The categories are the following:

1. English grammar: they all say it's so simple and yet nobody gets it right.
2. Misnomers and false friends.
3. Common basic mistakes.

English Grammar

Each nationality has its own black spots. Inevitably all speakers gain their own reputation too, in this cruel world of ours. The problem is that when you start learning English, there are all these big smiles telling you: "On the one hand pronunciation is difficult but on the other hand grammar is so easy."

Well, here is where it all begins: yes, English grammar is simple, true. The problem is that English is a language with very strict rules for word order, use of prepositions, etc. There is not as much room for improvisation when it comes to making up a sentence. Each verb is to be followed by one and only one preposition, otherwise it would mean something not only entirely, but also embarrassingly, different:

* Thank you very much for *putting me up* for the night (letting me stay).
* Thank you for *putting up with me* for the night (tolerate my presence).

In short, when speaking in English, a foreigner has to make a conscious effort to remember the cast-iron rules and avoid creating his/her own spur-of-the-moment version of the sentence structure.

Where do we always fail then? There are certain grammatical rules that tend to be overlooked by lecturers. Here you will find some examples of how to avoid frequently made mistakes:

* Never use the article *the* when the noun refers to something generic:
  – Peak concentration of the drug was measured on (the) *day 28*.
  – *Smoking* is undoubtedly *a* (the) risk factor.
* There are certain verbs that *always* need a specific preposition:
  – We listen *to* our patients.
  – Put *on* your coat and attend *to* the next patient.
  – Could you please explain *to* me how the accident happened.
* There are certain verbs that *will never ever* take a preposition:
  – You *must* take this tablet once a day.
  – If I were you I would *attend* the meeting.
* English structure is usually simpler than the grammar of your mother tongue. So, when speaking English, think in terms of: subject (S) + verb (V) + object (O):
  – The diagnosis (S) was (V) pneumonia (O).

The list of examples could be much longer. We do not intend this to be an exhaustive list; on the contrary, we encourage you with the help of Unit II and grammar manuals to find out your personal danger zones and create your personal grammar checklist.

Our advice is that whenever you are to give a talk in English, make sure a native English speaker, preferably a doctor, listens to you. Only such a listener will spot those sometimes silly and sometimes subtle grammatical mistakes that we always make and seem to follow us wherever we go. The rehearsal of your lecture before your native English speaker will always add value and spontaneity to your presentation.

Misnomers and False Friends

Every tongue has its own false friends. A thorough review of false friends is beyond the scope of this manual and we suggest that you look for those tricky names that sound similar in your language and in English but have completely different meanings.

Think, for example, about the term *graft versus host disease*. The translation of *host* has not been correct in some romance languages, and in Spanish the term *host*, which in this context means recipient, has been translated as *huésped* which means *person staying in another's house*. Many Spanish medical students have problems with the understanding of this disease because of the terminology used. Taking into account that what actually happens is that the graft reacts against the recipient, if the disease had been named *graft versus recipient disease*, the concept would probably be more precisely conveyed.

So from now on, identify false friends in your own language and make a list beginning with those belonging to your specialty; there is no use in knowing false friends in a language different from yours.

Medicine is full of misnomers. Think for a moment about the term *superficial femoral vein*. It is difficult to explain how a superficial femoral vein clot is actually in the deep venous system.

Many radiologists and oncologists all over the world say *normal mediastinal lymphadenopathy*. Lymphadenopathy means, from an etymological point of view, abnormal lymph node. A *normal lymphadenopathy* is as absurd as a *normal psychopathy*.

Etymologically *pancreas* means *all meat*, but there is no muscle at all in that endocrine and exocrine gland.

Etymologically *azygos* means *odd* which puts *hemiazygos* in a strange situation taking into consideration that odd numbers are not divisible by two.

The term *innominate vein* is as absurd as naming a baby *unnamed*.

When talking about false friends, very often we find that the real problem is the pronunciation. So we think it is just about time to get down to talking about one of our most dreaded nightmares: English phonetics. This is just not made for us. We all agree we are facing a tricky business here and, if given the choice, any physician in his/her right senses would prefer to read 100 or even a 1000 pages of English text rather than face the challenge of a one-minute conversation in the same language. Many well-trained professionals who have no speech impairment in their native tongue and can read English and understand it, the minute they are asked a very simple question in English, start shaking, frowning, stuttering, looking upwards as if calling for help from above, and finally after a few minutes they eventually say: "I don't know!".

We recommend that you should:

1. Not be afraid of sounding different or funny: English sounds *are* different and funny.
2. Enjoy the effort of using a different set of muscles in the mouth. In the beginning the "English muscles" may become stiff and even hurt, but persevere, it's only a sign of hard work.
3. Not worry about having in the beginning a broad or even embarrassing accent: it doesn't matter as long as you are understood. The idea is to communicate, to say what you think or feel, and not to give a performance in speech therapy.
4. Try to pronounce English words properly. As time goes by and you begin to feel relatively confident about your English, we encourage you to progressively and thoroughly study English phonetics. Bear in mind that if you keep your pronunciation as it was at the beginning you will sound like American or British people do when speaking with their unmistakable accent.
5. Rehearse standard collocations in both conversational and professional scenarios. Saying straightforward things such as "Do you know what I mean?" or "Would you do me a favor?" will provide you with extremely useful fluency tools.

Having your own *subtle* national accent in English is not a serious problem as long as the presentation conveys the correct message. However, as far as pronunciation is concerned, there are several tricky words that cannot be properly named false friends and need some extra attention:

In English there are some words that are spelt differently but sound very much the same. Consider the following, for example:

- *Ileum:* the distal portion of the small intestine, extending from the jejunum to the cecum.
- *Ilium:* the uppermost and widest of the three sections of the hip bone.

Imagine for a moment how surrealist it would be for our surgeons to mix up the bowel with the hip bone. Well, I suppose you could say it could be worse – at least both anatomical structures are roughly in the same area!

Again, consider the following:

The English word tear means two different things according to how we pronounce it:

- If tear [tiar] is pronounced[1], we mean the watery secretion of the lacrymal glands which serves to moisten the conjunctiva.

---

[1] For simplicity, the authors have taken the liberty of using an approximate representation of the pronunciation instead of using the phonetic signs. Apologies presented to our linguist colleagues who may have preferred a more orthodox transcription.

- If tear [tear] is pronounced, we are referring to the action of wounding or injuring, especially by ripping apart.

Common Basic Mistakes

These are some of the most common mistakes made in presentations at international congresses:

- 22-years-old man presenting ...
- *There was not biopsy* of the lesion
- It *allows to distinguish* between ...
- *Hemorrhagic tumors* can cause ...
- *The main group* of myxoid tumors *are* ...
- Could you tell me how old *is the patient*?
- Most of the times hemangiomas ...
- Looking forward to *hear* from you
- *Best* regards
- Are you suffering from *paresthesias*?
- There are multiple *metastasis*

***22-years-old* man presenting.** Many times the first sentence of the first slide of the presentation contains the first error. For those lecturers with an intermediate level this simple mistake is so evident that they barely believe it is one of the most frequent mistakes ever made.

It is quite obvious that the adjective *22-year-old* cannot be written in the plural and it should be written:

- 22-year-old man presenting.

***There was not biopsy* of the lesion.** This is a frequent and relatively subtle mistake made by upper-intermediate speakers. If you still prefer the use of the negative form you should say:

- There was not *any* biopsy of the lesion.

But the affirmative form is:

- There was no biopsy of the lesion.

***It allows to distinguish* between.** Two alternative sentences can be chosen:

- It allows us to distinguish between.
or
- It allows the distinction between.

***Haemorrhagic tumors* can cause.** Check your paper or presentation in order to avoid inconsistency in terms of American and British English.

This example shows a sentence made up of an American English word (*tumors*) and a British English word (*haemorrhagic*). So choose American or British spelling depending on the journal or congress you are sending your paper to.

Therefore, the sentence should read:

- *Haemorrhagic tumours* can cause.

or

- *Hemorrhagic tumors* can cause.

The main group of myxoid tumors are. Although extremely simple, this is one of the most frequent mistakes found in published medical papers.

Do not ever forget that in this kind of sentence, noun phrases are always in the singular and must be followed by the verb in the third person singular.

Noun phrase-verb lack of congruency is more likely to appear in long sentences, so try to avoid such sentences and when they are used check and double-check them carefully.

As everybody knows, but many forget in papers, the sentence should be:

- *The main group* of myxoid tumors *is*.

Could you tell me how old *is the patient*. Embedded questions are always troublesome. Whenever a question is embedded in another interrogative sentence its word order changes. This happens when, trying to be polite, we incorrectly change *What time is it?* to *Would you please tell me what time is it?* instead of to *Would you please tell me what time it is?*

In medicine, the direct question *How old is the patient?* must be transformed to its embedded form as follows:

- Could you tell me *how old the patient is*?

Most of the times hemangiomas. You can say *many times* but not *most of the times*. *Most of the time* is correct and you can use *commonly* or *frequently* as equivalent terms. Say instead:

- *Most of the time* hemangiomas.

Looking forward *to hear* from you. This a very frequent mistake at the end of formal letters such as those sent to editors. The mistake is based upon a grammatical error. *To* may be either a part of the infinitive or a preposition. In this case *to* is not a part of the infinitive of the verb *hear* but a part of the prepositional verb *look forward*; it is indeed a preposition.

There may be irreparable consequences of making this mistake. If you are trying to have an article published in a prestigious magazine you cannot make formal mistakes which can preclude the reading of your otherwise interesting article.

So instead of *looking forward to hear from you*, you should write:

* *Looking forward to hearing from you.*

Best regards. Although it is used in both academic and informal correspondence *best regards* is a mixture of two strong English collocations: *kind regards* and *best wishes*. In our opinion instead of *best regards*, which is colloquially acceptable, you should write:

* *Kind regards*

or simply

* *Regards*

Are you suffering from *paresthesia*? Many doctors forget that patients are not colleagues and use medical terminology which cannot be understood by them. This technical question would have been easily understood by saying:

* *Do you have pins and needles?*

There are multiple *metastasis*. Whenever you use a Latin term check its singular and plural. Metastasis is singular whereas metastases is plural so that *there are multiple metastasis* is not correct (see Unit VI). In this case, you should write:

* There are multiple *metastases.*

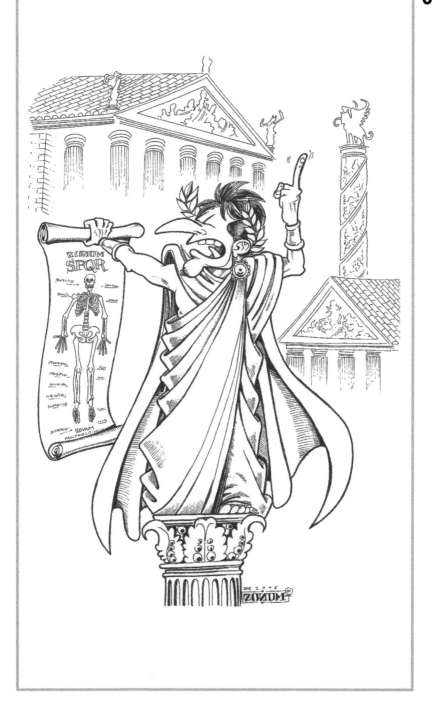

Unit VI Latin and Greek Terminology

Introduction

Latin and Greek terminology is another obstacle to be overcome on our way to becoming fluent in medical English. Romance-language speakers (Spanish, French, Italian ...) are undoubtedly at an advantage, although this advantage in theory can become a great drawback in terms of pronunciation and, particularly, in the use of the plural forms of Latin and Greek.

This unit is made up of a set of somewhat intuitive plural rules, several exercises containing Latin and Greek terminology, and finally a double list of Latin and Greek terms, the first one consisting of terms without English equivalents and the second one made up of terms with English equivalents.

Plural Rules

It is obvious that it is far from our intention to replace medical dictionaries and Latin or Greek text books. Conversely, this unit is aimed at giving some tips related to Latin and Greek terminology that can provide an intuitive approach to this challenging topic.

Our first piece of advice on this subject is that whenever you write a Latin or Greek word, firstly, check its spelling and, secondly, if the word you want to write is a plural one, never make it up. Although guessing the plural form could be acceptable as an exercise in itself, double-check the word by looking it up in a medical dictionary.

The following plural rules are useful to at least give us self-confidence in the use of usual Latin or Greek terms such as *metastasis – metastases, pelvis – pelves, bronchus – bronchi,* etc ...

Some overseas doctors do think that *metastasis* and *metastases* are equivalent terms, and they are absolutely wrong; the difference between a unique liver metastasis and multiple liver metastases is so obvious that no additional comments are needed.

There are many Latin and Greek words whose singular forms are almost never used as well as Latin and Greek terms whose plural forms are seldom said or written. Let us think, for example, about the singular form of *viscera* (*viscus*). Very few physicians are aware that liver is a *viscus* whereas liver and spleen are *viscera*. From a colloquial standpoint this discussion might be considered futile, but those who write papers do know that Latin/Greek terminology is always a nightmare and needs thorough revision, and that terms seldom used on a day-to-day basis have to be properly written in a scientific article. Again, let us consider the plural form of *pelvis* (*pelves*). To talk about several pelves is so rare that many doctors have never wondered what the plural form of pelvis is.

Although there are some exceptions, the following intuitive rules can be helpful with plural terms:

- Words ending in *-us* change to *-i*:
  - *Bronchus – bronchi*
- Words ending in *-um* change to *-a*:
  - *Acetabulum – acetabula*
- Words ending in *-a* change to *-ae*:
  - *Vena – venae*
- Words ending in *-ma* change to *-mata* or *-mas*:
  - *Sarcoma – sarcomata/sarcomas*
- Words ending in *-is* change to *-es*:
  - *Metastasis – metastases*
- Words ending in *-is* change to *-ides*:
  - *Arthritis – arthritides*
- Words ending in *-x* change to *-ces*:
  - *Pneumothorax – pneumothoraces*
- Words ending in *-cyx* change to *-cyges*:
  - *Coccyx – coccyges*
- Words ending in *-ion* change to *-ia*:
  - *Criterion – criteria*

Exercises

These quite simple exercises have been created with the purpose of encouraging you to become familiar with Latin and Greek plurals. From now on you should create your own exercises using your specialty's most common Latin and Greek terms.

1. There are two mistakes in the next paragraph. Find them:
   - The spleen is probably the least-studied abdominal viscera. Multiple metastasis are relatively uncommon.
   - (Viscus. Metastases)
2. Are there any mistakes in the next line?
   - Each leg has two menisci.
   - (No)

3. Are there any mistakes in the next line?
    - The patient's right knee had got lesions in its two meniscus.
    - (Yes. Menisci instead of meniscus)
4. How many mistakes can you find in the next paragraph?
    - Two thrombus were removed through mechanical aspiration. Although a third thrombi was detected, it was not removed.
    - (Two. Thrombi. Thrombus)
5. Is there any mistake in the next line?
    - Two iliofemoral thromboses were identified.
    - (No)
6. Write the plural form of cervix.
    - (Cervices)
7. Identify the mistakes:
    - Both superior and inferior veni cavi were occluded.
    - (Venae cavae)
8. Is the following sentence correct?
    - The only diagnostic criteria was fever.
    - (No. Criterion)
9. Any mistakes here?
    - Several metastasis were found in the liver.
    - (Metastases)
10. Is this correct?
    - Both humerus were shorter than normal.
    - (Humeri)

List of Latin and Greek Terms and Their Plurals

A
- **Acetabulum** pl. **Acetabula**. Cotyle
- **Acinus** pl. **Acini**. Acinus
- **Aditus** pl. **Aditus**. Aditus (entrance to a cavity)
  - Aditus ad antrum
  - Aditus ad aqueductum cerebri
  - Aditus ad infundibulum
  - Aditus ad saccum peritonaei minorum
  - Aditus glottidis inferior
- **Agger** pl. **Aggeres**. Agger (prominence)
  - Agger nasi
  - Agger perpendicularis
  - Agger valvae venae
- **Alveolus** pl. **Alveoli**. Alveolus
- **Alveus** pl. **Alvei**. Alveus (canal or cavity)
- **Amoeba** pl. **Amoebae**. Ameba
- **Ampulla** pl. **Ampullae**. Ampoule

- **Anastomosis** pl. **Anastomoses.** Anastomosis
- **Ansa** pl. **Ansae.** Loop
- **Antrum** pl. **Antra.** Antrum
- **Anus** pl. **Anus.** Anus
- **Aorta** pl. **Aortae.** Aorta
- **Apex** pl. **Apices.** Apex
- **Aphtha** pl. **Aphthae.** Aphtha (small ulcer)
- **Aponeurosis** pl. **Aponeuroses.** Aponeurosis
- **Apophysis** pl. **Apophyses.** Apophysis
- **Apparatus** pl. **Apparatus.** Apparatus (system)
- **Appendix** pl. **Appendices.** Appendage
- **Area** pl. **Areae.** Area
- **Areola** pl. **Areolae.** Areola
- **Arrector** pl. **Arrectores.** Erector
- **Arteria** pl. **Arteriae.** Artery
- **Arteriola** pl. **Arteriolae.** Arteriola (small artery)
- **Arthritis** pl. **Arthritides.** Arthritis
- **Articulatio** pl. **Articulationes.** Joint
- **Auricula** pl. **Auriculae.** Auricula (ear flap)
- **Auris** pl. **Aures.** Auris (ear)

B
- **Bacillus** pl. **Bacilli.** Stick-shape bacterium
- **Bacterium** pl. **Bacteria.** Bacterium
- **Borborygmus** pl. **Borborygmi.** Borborygmus (gastrointestinal sound related to the passage of gas)
- **Brachium** pl. **Brachia.** Arm
- **Bronchium** pl. **Bronchia.** Bronchus
- **Bronchus** pl. **Bronchi.** Bronchus
- **Bulla** pl. **Bullae.** Bulla
- **Bursa** pl. **Bursae.** Bursa (bag)

C
- **Calcaneus** pl. **Calcanei.** Calcaneus
- **Calculus** pl. **Calculi.** Stone
- **Calix** pl. **Calices.** Calix
- **Calx** pl. **Calces.** Heel
- **Canalis** pl. **Canales.** Canal
- **Cancellus** pl. **Cancelli.** Reticulum
- **Cancrum** pl. **Cancra.** Cancrum (gangrene)
  - Cancrum nasi
- **Capillus** pl. **Capilli.** Hair
- **Capitulum** pl. **Capitula.** Condyle
- **Caput** pl. **Capita.** Head
- **Carcinoma** pl. **Carcinomas** (or **Carcinomata**). Carcinoma (cancer)
- **Carina** pl. **Carinae.** Carina (tracheal carina)

- **Cartilago** pl. **Cartilagines.** Cartilage
- **Cauda** pl. **Caudae.** Tail
- **Caverna** pl. **Cavernae.** Cavern
- **Cavitas** pl. **Cavitates.** Cavity
- **Cella** pl. **Cellae.** Cell
- **Centrum** pl. **Centra.** Center
- **Cerebrum** pl. **Cerebra.** Brain
- **Cervix** pl. **Cervices.** Cervix (uterine cervix)
- **Chiasma** pl. **Chiasmata.** Chiasm
- **Choana** pl. **Choanae.** Choana
- **Chorda** pl. **Chordae.** String
- **Cicatrix** pl. **Cicatrices.** Scar
- **Cilium** pl. **Cilia.** Cilium
- **Cingulum** pl. **Cingula.** Cingulum (belt-shaped structure)
- **Cisterna** pl. **Cisternae.** Cistern
- **Claustrum** pl. **Claustra.** Claustrum
- **Clitoris** pl. **Clitorides.** Clitoris
- **Clivus** pl. **Clivi.** Clivus
- **Clostridium** pl. **Clostridia.** Clostridium
- **Coccus** pl. **Cocci.** Coccus (rounded bacterium)
- **Coccyx** pl. **Coccyges.** Coccyx
- **Cochlea** pl. **Cochleae.** Cochlea
- **Comedo** pl. **Comedones.** Comedo
- **Concha** pl. **Conchae.** Concha (shell-shaped structure)
- **Condyloma** pl. **Condylomata.** Condyloma (condyloma acuminatum)
- **Conjunctiva** pl. **Conjunctivae.** Conjunctiva
- **Cor** pl. **Corda.** Heart
- **Corium** pl. **Coria.** Dermis
- **Cornu** pl. **Cornua.** Horn
- **Corona** pl. **Coronae.** Corona (crown)
- **Corpus** pl. **Corpora.** Body
- **Corpusculum** pl. **Corpuscula.** Corpuscle
- **Cortex** pl. **Cortices.** Cortex
- **Coxa** pl. **Coxae.** Hip
- **Cranium** pl. **Crania.** Skull
- **Crisis** pl. **Crises.** Crisis
- **Criterion** pl. **Criteria.** Criterion
- **Crus** pl. **Crura.** Leg
- **Crusta** pl. **Crustae.** Crust, scab
- **Crypta** pl. **Cryptae.** Crypt
- **Cubitus** pl. **Cubiti.** Cubitus (ulna)
- **Culmen** pl. **Culmina.** Culmen (cerebellar lobe)

D

- Decussatio pl. **Decussationes**. Decussation
- Dens pl. **Dentes**. Tooth pl. Teeth
- Dermatitis pl. **Dermatitides**. Dermatitis
- Dermatosis pl. **Dermatoses**. Dermatosis
- Diaphragma pl. **Diaphragmata**. Diaphragm
- Diaphysis pl. **Diaphyses**. Shaft
- Diarthrosis pl. **Diarthroses**. Diarthrosis
- Diastema pl. **Diastemata**. Diastema (congenital fissure)
- Diverticulum pl. **Diverticula**. Diverticulum
- Dorsum pl. **Dorsa**. Back
- Ductus pl. **Ductus**. Duct
- Duodenum pl. **Duodena**. Duodenum

E

- Ecchymosis pl. **Ecchymoses**. Ecchymosis
- Effluvium pl. **Effluvia**. Effluvium (fall)
- Encephalitis pl. **Encephalitides**. Encephalitis
- Endocardium pl. **Endocardia**. Endocardium
- Endometrium pl. **Endometria**. Endometrium
- Endothelium pl. **Endothelia**. Endothelium
- Epicondylus pl. **Epicondyli**. Epicondylus
- Epidermis pl. **Epidermides**. Epidermis
- Epididymis pl. **Epididymes**. Epididymis
- Epiphysis pl. **Epiphyses**. Epiphysis
- Epithelium pl. **Epithelia**. Epithelium
- Esophagus pl. **Esophagi**. Esophagus
- Exostosis pl. **Exostoses**. Exostosis

F

- Facies pl. **Facies**. Face
- Falx pl. **Falces**. Falx (sickle-shaped structure)
- Fascia pl. **Fasciae**. Fascia
- Fasciculus pl. **Fasciculi**. Fasciculus
- Femur pl. **Femora**. Femur
- Fenestra pl. **Fenestrae**. Fenestra (window)
- Fetus pl. **Feti**. Fetus
- Fibra pl. **Fibrae**. Fiber
- Filamentum pl. **Filamenta**. Filament
- Filaria pl. **Filariae**. Filaria
- Filum pl. **Fila**. Filum
- Fimbria pl. **Fimbriae**. Fimbria (stripe-shaped structure)
- Flagellum pl. **Flagella**. Flagellum (whip-like locomotory organelle)
- Flexura pl. **Flexurae**. Flexure
- Folium pl. **Folia**. Folium (leaf-shaped structure)
- Folliculus pl. **Folliculi**. Follicle

- Foramen pl. **Foramina**. Foramen (hole)
- Formula pl. **Formulae**. Formula
- Fornix pl. **Fornices**. Fornix (arch-shaped structure)
- Fossa pl. **Fossae**. Fossa
- Fovea pl. **Foveae**. Fovea
- Frenulum pl. **Frenula**. Frenulum
- Fungus pl. **Fungi**. Fungus
- Funiculus pl. **Funiculi**. Cord
- Furfur pl. **Furfures**. Dandruff
- Furunculus pl. **Furunculi**. Furuncle

G

- Ganglion pl. **Ganglia**. Node
- Geniculum pl. **Genicula**. Geniculum (knee-shaped structure)
- Genu pl. **Genua**. Knee
- Genus pl. **Genera**. Genus
- Gestosis pl. **Gestoses**. Gestosis (pregnancy impairment)
- Gingiva pl. **Gingivae**. Gum
- Glandula pl. **Glandulae**. Gland
- Glans pl. **Glandes**. Glans
- Globus pl. **Globi**. Globus
- Glomerulus pl. **Glomeruli**. Glomerulus
- Glomus pl. **Glomera**. Glomus
- Glottis pl. **Glottides**. Glottis
- Gonion pl. **Gonia**. Gonion
- Granulatio pl. **Granulationes**. Granulatio
- Gumma pl. **Gummata**. Gumma
- Gutta pl. **Guttae**. Gout
- Gyrus pl. **Gyri**. Convolution

H

- Hallux pl. **Halluces**. Hallux (first toe)
- Hamulus pl. **Hamuli**. Hook
- Haustrum pl. **Haustra**. Haustrum
- Hiatus pl. **Hiatus**. Hiatus
- Hilum pl. **Hila**. Hilum
- Hircus pl. **Hirci**. Hircus (armpit hair, also armpit smell)
- Humerus pl. **Humeri**. Humerus
- Humor pl. **Humores**. Humor (fluid)
- Hypha pl. **Hyphae**. Hypha

I

- Ilium pl. **Ilia**. Iliac bone
- Incisura pl. **Incisurae**. Incisure
- Incus pl. **Incudes**. Incus (anvil)
- Index pl. **Indices**. Index (second finger)

- **Indusium** pl. **Indusia.** Indusium (membrane)
- **Infundibulum** pl. **Infundibula.** Infundibulum
- **Insula** pl. **Insulae.** Insula
- **Intersectio** pl. **Intersectiones.** Intersection
- **Interstitium** pl. **Interstitia.** Interstice
- **Intestinum** pl. **Intestina.** Bowel
- **Iris** pl. **Irides.** Iris
- **Ischium** pl. **Ischia.** Ischium
- **Isthmus** pl. **Isthmi.** Isthmus

J

- **Jugum** pl. **Juga.** Yoke
- **Junctura** pl. **Juncturae.** Joint

L

- **Labium** pl. **Labia.** Lip
- **Labrum** pl. **Labra.** Lip
- **Lacuna** pl. **Lacunae.** Lacuna (pond)
- **Lamellipodium** pl. **Lamellipodia.** Lamellipodium
- **Lamina** pl. **Laminae.** Layer
- **Larva** pl. **Larvae.** Larva
- **Larynx** pl. **Larynges.** Larynx
- **Latus** pl. **Latera.** Flank
- **Lemniscus** pl. **Lemnisci.** Lemniscus
- **Lentigo** pl. **Lentigines.** Lentigo
- **Lienculus** pl. **Lienculi.** Lienculus (accessory spleen)
- **Ligamentum** pl. **Ligamenta.** Ligament
- **Limbus** pl. **Limbi.** Limbus (border)
- **Limen** pl. **Limina.** Threshold
- **Linea** pl. **Lineae.** Line
- **Lingua** pl. **Linguae.** Tongue
- **Lingula** pl. **Lingulae.** Lingula
- **Lipidosis** pl. **Lipidoses.** Lipidosis
- **Liquor** pl. **Liquores.** Fluid
- **Lobulus** pl. **Lobuli.** Lobule
- **Lobus** pl. **Lobi.** Lobe
- **Loculus** pl. **Loculi.** Loculus (cavity or small chamber)
- **Locus** pl. **Loci.** Locus (place)
- **Lumbus** pl. **Lumbi.** Lumbus
- **Lumen** pl. **Lumina.** Lumen
- **Lunula** pl. **Lunulae.** Lunula
- **Lymphonodus** pl. **Lymphonodi.** Lymph node

M

- Macula pl. **Maculae.** Macula (stain)
- Malleollus pl. **Malleoli.** Malleollus
- Malleus pl. **Mallei.** Malleus (hammer)
- Mamilla pl. **Mamillae.** Mamilla
- Mamma pl. **Mammae.** Breast
- Mandibula pl. **Mandibulae.** Jaw
- Manubrium pl. **Manubria.** Manubrium (handle)
- Manus pl. **Manus.** Hand
- Margo pl. **Margines.** Margin
- Matrix pl. **Matrices.** Matrix (tooth matrix, nail matrix)
- Maxilla pl. **Maxillae.** Maxilla
- Meatus pl. **Meatus.** Meatus (canal)
- Medium pl. **Media.** Medium (i.e. culture medium)
- Medulla pl. **Medullae.** Marrow
- Membrana pl. **Membranae.** Membrane
- Membrum pl. **Membra.** Limb
- Meningitis pl. **meningitides.** Meningitis
- Meningococcus pl. **Meningococci.** Meningococcus
- Meninx pl. **Meninges.** Meninx
- Mentum pl. **Menti.** Chin
- Mesocardium pl. **Mesocardia.** Mesocardium
- Mesonephros pl. **Mesonephroi.** Mesonephros
- Mesothelium pl. **Mesothelia.** Mesothelium
- Mesovarium pl. **Mesovaria.** Mesovaium
- Metacarpus pl. **Metacarpi.** Metacarpus
- Metanephros pl. **Metanephroi.** Metanephros
- Metaphysis pl. **Metaphyses.** Metaphysis
- Metastasis pl. **Metastases.** Metastasis
- Metatarsus pl. **Metatarsi.** Metatarsus
- Microvillus pl. **Microvilli.** Microvillus
- Mitochondrion pl. **Mitochondria.** Mitochondrion
- Mitosis pl. **Mitoses.** Mitosis
- Modiolus pl. **Modioli.** Modiolus (cochlear modiolus)
- Mons pl. **Montes.** Mons (mount)
- Mors pl. **Mortes.** Death
- Mucolipidosis pl. **Mucolipidoses.** Mucolipidosis
- Mucro pl. **Mucrones.** Mucro, e.g., mucro sterni (sharp-tipped structure)
- Musculus pl. **Musculi.** Muscle
- Mycelium pl. **Mycelia.** Mycelium
- Mycoplasma pl. **Mycoplasmata.** Mycoplasma
- Myocardium pl. **Myocardia.** Myocardium
- Myocomma pl. **Myocommata.** Myocomma
- Myofibrilla pl. **Myofibrillae.** Myofibrilla
- Myomitochondrion pl. **Myomitochondria.** Myomitochondrion
- Myrinx pl. **Myringes.** Myrinx (eardrum)

N

- **Naris** pl. **Nares.** Naris (nasal fossa)
- **Nasus** pl. **Nasi.** Nose
- **Nebula** pl. **Nebulae.** Nebula (corneal nebula)
- **Neisseria** pl. **Neisseriae.** Neisseria
- **Nephritis** pl. **Nephritides.** Nephritis
- **Nervus** pl. **Nervi.** Nerve
- **Neuritis** pl. **Neuritides.** Neuritis
- **Neurosis** pl. **Neuroses.** Neurosis
- **Nevus** pl. **Nevi.** Nevus
- **Nidus** pl. **Nidi.** Nidus (nest)
- **Nodulus** pl. **Noduli.** Nodule
- **Nucleolus** pl. **Nucleoli.** Nucleolus
- **Nucleus** pl. **Nuclei.** Nucleus

O

- **Occiput** pl. **Occipitis.** Occiput
- **Oculentum** pl. **Oculenta.** Eye ointment
- **Oculus** pl. **Oculi.** Eye
- **Oliva** pl. **Olivae.** Rounded elevation
- **Omentum** pl. **Omenta.** Peritoneal fold
- **Oogonium** pl. **Oogonia.** Oocyte
- **Operculum** pl. **Opercula.** Operculum
- **Organum** pl. **Organa.** Organ
- **Orificium** pl. **Orificia.** Opening
- **Os** pl. **Orae.** Mouth
- **Os** pl. **Ossa.** Bone
- **Ossiculum** pl. **Ossicula.** Ossicle
- **Ostium** pl. **Ostia.** Opening into a tubular organ
- **Ovarium** pl. **Ovaria.** Ovary
- **Ovulum** pl. **Ovula.** Ovule

P

- **Palatum** pl. **palati.** Palate
- **Palma** pl. **Palmae.** Palm
- **Palpebra** pl. **Palpebrae.** Eyelid
- **Paralysis** pl. **Paralyses.** Palsy
- **Paries** pl. **Parietes.** Wall
- **Pars** pl. **Partes.** Part
- **Pectus** pl. **Pectora.** Chest
- **Pes** pl. **Pedes.** Foot
- **Pilula** pl. **Pilulae.** Pill
- **Planum** pl. **Plana.** Plane
- **Plica** pl. **Plicae.** Fold
- **Pollex** pl. **Pollices.** Thumb
- **Polus** pl. **Poli.** Pole

- **Portio** pl. **Portiones.** Portion
- **Porus** pl. **Pori.** Pore
- **Pulmo** pl. **Pulmones.** Lung
- **Punctum** pl. **Puncta.** Point
- **Pancreas** pl. **Pancreata.** Pancreas
- **Panniculus** pl. **Panniculi.** Panniculus
- **Pannus** pl. **Panni.** Pannus
- **Papilla** pl. **Papillae.** Papilla
- **Paradidymis** pl. **Paradidymides.** Paradidymis
- **Paraganglion** pl. **Paraganglia.** Paraganglion
- **Parametrium** pl. **Parametria.** Parametrium
- **Paranephros** pl. **Paranephroi.** Paranephros (adrenal)
- **Paraproctium** pl. **Paraproctia.** Paraproctium
- **Patagium** pl. **Patagia.** Patagium
- **Patella** pl. **Patellae.** Patella
- **Pediculus** pl. **Pediculi.** Pediculus
- **Pedunculus** pl. **Pedunculi.** Pedunculus
- **Pelvis** pl. **Pelves.** Pelvis
- **Pericardium** pl. **Pericardia.** Pericardium
- **Perikaryon** pl. **Perikarya.** Perikaryon
- **Perikyma** pl. **Perikymata.** Perikyma
- **Perimetrium** pl. **Perimetria.** Perimetrium
- **Perimysium** pl. **Perimysia.** Perimysium
- **Perineum** pl. **Perinea.** Perineum
- **Perineurium** pl. **Perineuria.** Perineurium
- **Periodontium** pl. **Periodontia.** Periodontium
- **Perionychium** pl. **Perionychia.** Perionychium
- **Periosteum** pl. **Periostea.** Periosteum
- **Periostosis** pl. **Periostoses.** Periostosis
- **Perithelium** pl. **Perithelia.** Perithelium
- **Peritoneum** pl. **Peritonea.** Peritoneum
- **Petechia** pl. **Petechiae.** Petechia
- **Phalanx** pl. **Phalanges.** Phalanx
- **Phallus** pl. **Phalli.** Phallus
- **Pharynx** pl. **Pharynges.** Pharynx
- **Phenomenon** pl. **Phenomena.** Phenomenon
- **Philtrum** pl. **Philtra.** Philtrum
- **Phimosis** pl. **Phimoses.** Phimosis
- **Phlyctena** pl. **Phlyctenae.** Phlyctena
- **Phlyctenula** pl. **Phlyctenulae.** Phlyctenule
- **Pia mater.** Pia mater
- **Planta** pl. **Plantae.** Planta
- **Platysma** pl. **Platysmata.** Platysma
- **Plexus** pl. **Plexuses.** Plexus
- **Pneumoconiosis** pl. **Pneumoconioses.** Pneumoconiosis
- **Pons** pl. **Pontes.** Pons

- **Porion** pl. **Poria**. Porium
- **Porta** pl. **Portae**. Porta
- **Preputium** pl. **Preputia**. Preputium
- **Princeps** pl. **Principes**. Princeps
- **Processus** pl. **Processus**. Processus
- **Prominentia** pl. **Prominentiae**. Prominentia
- **Promontorium** pl. **Promontoria**. Promontorium
- **Pronephros** pl. **Pronephroi**. Pronephros
- **Prophylaxis** pl. **Prophylaxes**. Prophylaxis
- **Prosthesis** pl. **Prostheses**. Prosthesis
- **Psalterium** pl. **Psalteria**. Psalterium
- **Pseudopodium** pl. **Pseudopodia**. Pseudopodium
- **Psychosis** pl. **Psychoses**. Psychosis
- **Ptosis** pl. **Ptoses**. Ptosis
- **Pubis** pl. **Pubes**. Pubis
- **Pudendum** pl. **Pudenda**. Pudendum
- **Puerpera** pl. **Puerperae**. Puerpera
- **Puerperium** pl. **Puerperia**. Puerperium
- **Pylorus** pl. **Pylori**. Pylorus

R

- **Rachis** pl. **Rachides**. Rachis
- **Radiatio** pl. **Radiationes**. Radiation
- **Radius** pl. **Radii**. Radius
- **Radix** pl. **Radices**. Root
- **Ramus** pl. **Rami**. Branch
- **Receptaculum** pl. **Receptacula**. Receptaculum
- **Recessus** pl. **Recessus**. Recess
- **Rectum** pl. **Recta**. Rectum
- **Regio** pl. **Regiones**. Region
- **Ren** pl. **Renes**. Kidney
- **Rete** pl. **Retia**. Network
- **Reticulum** pl. **Reticula**. Reticulum
- **Retinaculum** pl. **Retinacula**. Retinaculum
- **Rima** pl. **Rimae**. Rima
- **Rostrum** pl. **Rostra**. Rostrum
- **Ruga** pl. **Rugae**. Ridge

S

- **Sacculus** pl. **Sacculi**. Small pouch
- **Saccus** pl. **Sacci**. Pouch
- **Sacrum** pl. **Sacra**. Sacral bone
- **Salpinx** pl. **Salpinges**. Fallopian tube
- **Scapula** pl. **Scapulae**. Scapula
- **Sclerosis** pl. **Scleroses**. Sclerosis
- **Scolex** pl. **Scoleces**. Scolex

- Scotoma pl. **Scotomata.** Scotoma
- Scrotum pl. **Scrota.** Scrotum
- Scutulum pl. **Scutula.** Scutulum
- Scybalum pl. **Scybala.** Scybalum
- Segmentum pl. **Segmenta.** Segment
- Semen pl. **Semina.** Semen
- Sensorium pl. **Sensoria.** Sensorium
- Sepsis pl. **Sepses.** Sepsis
- Septum pl. **Septa.** Septum
- Sequela pl. **Sequelae.** Sequela
- Sequestrum pl. **Sequestra.** Sequestrum
- Serosa pl. **Serosae.** Serosa
- Serum pl. **Sera.** Serum
- Sinciput pl. **Sincipita.** Sinciput
- Sinus pl. **Sinus.** Sinus
- Spatium pl. **Spatia.** Space
- Spectrum pl. **Spectra.** Spectrum
- Spermatozoon pl. **Spermatozoa.** Spermatozoid
- Spiculum pl. **Spicula.** Spike
- Spina pl. **Spinae.** Spine
- Splenium pl. **Splenia.** Splenium
- Splenunculus pl. **Splenunculi.** Accessory spleen
- Sputum pl. **Sputa.** Sputum
- Squama pl. **Squamae.** Scale
- Stapes pl. **Stapes, Stapedes.** Stapes
- Staphylococcus pl. **Staphylococci.** Staphylococcus
- Stasis pl. **Stases.** Stasis
- Statoconium pl. **Statoconia.** Statoconium
- Stenosis pl. **Stenoses.** Stenosis
- Stereocilium pl. **Stereocilia.** Stereocilium
- Sternum pl. **Sterna.** Sternum
- Stigma pl. **Stigmata.** Stigma
- Stimulus pl. **Stimuli.** Stimulus
- Stoma pl. **Stomata.** Stoma
- Stratum pl. **Strata.** Stratum
- Stria pl. **Striae.** Fluting
- Stroma pl. **Stromata.** Stroma
- Struma pl. **Strumae.** Struma
- Subiculum pl. **Subicula.** Subiculum
- Substantia pl. **Substantiae.** Substance
- Sulcus pl. **Sulci.** Sulcus
- Supercilium pl. **Supercilia.** Eyebrow
- Sustentaculum pl. **Sustentacula.** Sustentaculum
- Sutura pl. **Suturae.** Suture
- Symphysis pl. **Symphyses.** Symphysis
- Synapse pl. **Synapses.** Synapse

- **Synchondrosis** pl. **Synchondroses.** Synchondrosis
- **Syncytium** pl. **Syncytia.** Syncytium
- **Syndesmosis** pl. **Syndesmoses.** Syndesmosis
- **Synechia** pl. **Synechiae.** Synechia
- **Syrinx** pl. **Syringes.** Syrinx

T

- **Talus** pl. **Tali.** Talus
- **Tarsus** pl. **Tarsi.** Tarsus
- **Tectum** pl. **Tecta.** Roof
- **Tegmen** pl. **Tegmina.** Roof
- **Tegmentum** pl. **Tegmenta.** Covering
- **Tela** pl. **Telae.** Membrane
- **Telangiectasis** pl. **Telangiectases.** Telangiectasis
- **Tenaculum** pl. **Tenacula.** Surgical clamp
- **Tendo** pl. **Tendines.** Tendon, sinew
- **Tenia** pl. **Teniae.** Tenia
- **Tentorium** pl. **Tentoria.** Tentorium
- **Teras** pl. **Terata.** Monster
- **Testis** pl. **Testes.** Testicle
- **Thalamus** pl. **Thalami.** Thalamus
- **Theca** pl. **Thecae.** Theca
- **Thelium** pl. **Thelia.** Nipple
- **Thesis** pl. **Theses.** Thesis
- **Thorax** pl. **Thoraces.** Chest
- **Thrombosis** pl. **Thromboses.** Thrombosis
- **Thrombus** pl. **Thrombi.** Thrombus
- **Thymus** pl. **Thymi.** Thymus
- **Tibia** pl. **Tibiae.** Tibia
- **Tonsilla** pl. **Tonsillae.** Tonsil
- **Tophus** pl. **Tophi.** Tophus
- **Torulus** pl. **Toruli.** Small papilla
- **Trabecula** pl. **Trabeculae.** Trabecula
- **Trachea** pl. **Tracheae.** Trachea
- **Tractus** pl. **Tractus.** Tract
- **Tragus** pl. **Tragi.** Tragus
- **Trapezium** pl. **Trapezia.** Trapezium bone
- **Trauma** pl. **Traumata.** Trauma
- **Trigonum** pl. **Trigona.** Trigonum
- **Trochlea** pl. **Trochleae.** Trochlea
- **Truncus** pl. **Trunci.** Trunk
- **Tuba** pl. **Tubae.** Tube
- **Tuberculum** pl. **Tubercula.** Tuberculum
- **Tubulus** pl. **Tubuli.** Small tube
- **Tunica** pl. **Tunicae.** Tunic

- **Turunda** pl. **Turundae.** Turunda
- **Tylosis** pl. **Tyloses.** Tylosis

U

- **Ulcus** pl. **Ulcera.** Ulcer
- **Ulna** pl. **Ulnae.** Ulna
- **Umbilicus** pl. **Umbilici.** Navel
- **Unguis** pl. **Ungues.** Nail
- **Uterus** pl. **Uteri.** Uterus
- **Utriculus** pl. **Utriculi.** Utriculus
- **Uveitis** pl. **Uveitides.** Uveítis
- **Uvula** pl. **Uvuli.** Uvula

V

- **Vagina** pl. **Vaginae.** Vagina
- **Vaginitis** pl. **Vaginitides.** Vaginitis
- **Vagus** pl. **Vagi.** Vagus nerve
- **Valva** pl. **Valvae.** Leaflet
- **Valvula** pl. **Valvulae.** Valve
- **Varix** pl. **Varices.** Varix
- **Vas** pl. **Vasa.** Vessel
- **Vasculum** pl. **Vascula.** Small vessel
- **Vena** pl. **Venae.** Vein
- **Ventriculus** pl. **Ventriculi.** Ventricle. Stomach
- **Venula** pl. **Venulae.** Venule
- **Vermis** pl. **Vermes.** Worm
- **Verruca** pl. **Verrucae.** Wart
- **Vertebra** pl. **vertebrae.** Vertebra
- **Vertex** pl. **Vertices.** Vertex
- **Vesica** pl. **Vesicae.** Bladder
- **Vesicula** pl. **Vesiculae.** Vesicle
- **Vestibulum** pl. **Vestibula.** Entrance to a cavity
- **Villus** pl. **Villi.** Villus
- **Vinculum** pl. **Vincula.** Band, band-like structure
- **Virus** pl. **Viruses.** Virus
- **Viscus** pl. **Viscera.** Viscus
- **Vitiligo** pl. **Vitiligines.** Vitiligo
- **Vomer** pl. **Vomeris.** Vomer bone
- **Vulva** pl. **Vulvae.** Vulva

Z

- **Zona** pl. **Zonae.** Zone
- **Zonula** pl. **Zonulae.** Small zone
- **Zygapophysis** pl. **Zygapophyses.** Vertebral articular apophysis

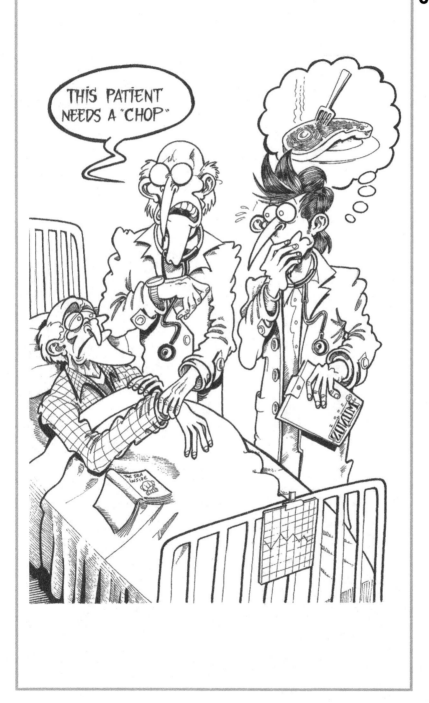

Unit VII Acronyms and Abbreviations

Introduction

"The patient went from the ER to the OR and then to the ICU."

It is an irrefutable fact that doctors' speech is full of abbreviations. Health-care professionals from both the Spanish- and English-speaking worlds use at least ten abbreviations per minute (this is our own home-made statistic; please don't quote us). This high prevalence has led us to consider medical abbreviations as a challenging pandemic.

There are several "types" of abbreviations, namely:

* Straightforward abbreviations
* Extra-nice abbreviations
* Expanded-term abbreviations
* Energy-saving abbreviations
* Double-meaning abbreviations
* Mind-blowing abbreviations

Let us begin with the nice ones; we call them the *straightforward* abbreviations because for each nice abbreviation in your own language there is a nice English equivalent. No beating around the bush here. It's just a matter of changing letter order, identifying the abbreviations and learning them. Let me give you a few examples so you can enjoy the simple things in life ... while you can!

HRT	Hormone replacement therapy
LVOT	Left ventricle outflow tract
ASD	Atrial septal defect
VSD	Ventricular septal defect
TEE	Transesophageal echocardiography
LDA	Left anterior descending artery
ACE	Angiotensin converting enzyme

There are other kinds of abbreviation: the *extra-nice* ones. They are mostly used for drugs or chemical substances whose name has three or four syllables too many. They are extra nice because they are usually the same in many languages. Let's see just an example:

- CPK   Creatine phosphokinase

In the next group, we have put together some examples of abbreviations that are widely used in English but that are generally preferred in their expanded form in other languages. Since language is an ever-changing creature, we are sure that these terms will eventually be abbreviated in many languages but so far you can hear them referred to mostly as expanded terms:

NSCLC   Non-small cell lung cancer
PBSC   Peripheral blood stem cell

There is another group which we call the *energy-saving* abbreviations. These are abbreviations that many languages leave in the English original and, of course, when expanding them the first letter of each word doesn't match the abbreviation. We call them energy-saving because it wouldn't have been so difficult to come up with a real "national" abbreviation for that term. When looking for examples, we realized that most hormone names are energy-saving abbreviations:

FSH   Follicle-stimulating hormone
TNF   Tumor necrosis factor
PAW   Pulmonary arterial wedge

There is yet another kind, which we call the *double-meaning* abbreviations. This is when one abbreviation can refer to two different terms. The context helps, of course, to discern the real meaning. However, it is worth keeping an eye open for these because, if misinterpreted, these abbreviations might get you into an embarrassing situation:

- PCR
  - Polymerase chain reaction
  - Plasma clearance tests
- HEV
  - Human enteric virus
  - Hepatitis E virus
- PID
  - Pelvic inflammatory disease
  - Prolapsed intervertebral disc
- CSF
  - Colony-stimulating factor
  - Cerebrospinal fluid

The funniest abbreviations are those that become acronyms in which the pronunciation resembles a word that has nothing to do with the abbreviation's meaning. We call this group the *mind-blowing* abbreviations.

A *cabbage* in English is that nice vegetable known for its gasogenic properties. However, when an English-speaking surgeon says "This patient is a clear candidate for *cabbage*", he/she isn't talking about what the patient should have for lunch, but rather the type of surgery he/she is suggesting should be performed. Thus, *cabbage* is the colloquial way of referring to *CABG* (coronary artery bypass grafting).

If you happen to be eavesdropping in a corridor and you hear an oncologist saying "I think your patient needs a *chop*", you walk on down the corridor, wondering whether this new alternative therapy will consist of a pork or a lamb chop. But then you quickly realize that the specialist you were spying on was actually referring to a *CHOP* (a regimen of cyclophosphamide, hydroxydaunomycin, oncovin and prednisone, used in cancer chemotherapy).

There are more abbreviations out there, and there are also more to come. The medical profession is sure to keep us busy catching up with its incursions into linguistic creation.

Regardless of the "type" of abbreviation you have before you, we will give you three pieces of advice:

1. Identify the most common abbreviations.
2. Read the abbreviations in your lists.
3. Review abbreviation lists on your specialty.

Identify the most common abbreviations. Identify the most common abbreviations in your specialty and in the hospital jargon and write them down in your own lists. For example, if you happen to be a radiologist, make a list of radiological abbreviations including terms such as CXR (chest X-ray) and UKB (ureter, kidneys and bladder), and a second list of abbreviations such as OR (operating room) and NICU (neonatal intensive care unit).

Read the abbreviations in your lists. Read the abbreviations in your lists in a natural way. Bear in mind that to be able to identify written abbreviations may not be enough. From this standpoint, there are three types of abbreviations:

1. Spelt abbreviations
2. Read abbreviations (acronyms)
3. Half-spelled/half-read abbreviations

Nobody would understand a spelt abbreviation if you read it and nobody would understand a read abbreviation if you spell it.

Let us make clear what we are trying to say with an example. LAM stands for lymphangiomyomatosis and must be read *lam*. Nobody would understand you if instead of saying *lam* you spell L-A-M. Therefore, never spell a "read abbreviation" and never read a "spelt abbreviation".

Most abbreviations are spelt abbreviations, and are usually those in which the letter order makes them almost impossible to read. Think, for example, of COPD (chronic obstructive pulmonary disease) and try to read the abbreviation instead of spelling it. Never use the "expanded form" (chronic obstructive pulmonary disease) of a classic abbreviation such as this one because it would sound extraordinarily unnatural.

Some abbreviations have become acronyms and therefore must be read and not spelt. Their letter order allows us to read them. LAM belongs to this group.

The third type is made up of abbreviations such as CPAP (continuous positive airway pressure) which is pronounced something like *C-pap*. If you spell out CPAP (C-P-A-P), nobody will understand you.

Review abbreviation lists on your specialty. Review as many abbreviation lists on your specialty as you can and double-check them until you are familiar with their meaning and pronunciation.

Common Sentences Containing Abbreviations

The following sections present sets of common sentences containing abbreviations, each set followed by the definitions of the abbreviations used in that set.

General

Sentences:

* A 40-year-old man visited our hospital, and was diagnosed as having Felty's syndrome because of splenomegaly and pancytopenia as well as definite RA.
* MCV, MCHC, LDH, ANA and RF values are normal.
* The platelet and WBC counts exceeded their normal ranges. He was diagnosed as suffering from ... (ITP, CMML, AML, CML). Two months after, he received a BMT.
* Foreign bodies display a variable signal intensity on both T1- and T2-weighted images. MR shows an inflammatory response while CT can show the retained foreign body. US evaluation could be useful in selected patients.
* COPD is a risk factor in the development of TB.
* Cholera can be diagnosed by the presence of CTX in stools.

- A 16-year-old female suffering from fever, chills, rash and presenting multiple nodular opacities in CXR was diagnosed as having ... (RMSF, BPF, DGI).
- An ECG was obtained, and showed ... (RBBB, LBBB, APCs, VPCs, AF, VF).
- He is actually under treatment with ACEI. Ten years ago he was treated with PTCA because of the three AMI he had suffered.
- RA and SSc are more common in females.
- PCP and PML are two of the complications that can be suffered by AIDS patients.
- Cutaneous manifestations of SLE can be divided into SCLE (acute) and DEL (chronic).

Definitions:

ACEI	Angiotensin-converting enzyme inhibitor
AF	Atrial fibrillation
AIDS	Acquired immunodeficiency syndrome
AMI	Acute myocardial infarction
AML	Acute myeloid leukemia
ANA	Antinuclear antibodies
APCs	Atrial premature complexes
BMT	Bone marrow transplantation
BPF	Brazilian purpuric fever
CML	Chronic myeloid leukemia
CMML	Chronic myelomonocytic leukemia
COPD	Chronic obstructive pulmonary disease
CT	Computed tomography
CTX	Cholera toxin
CXR	Chest X-ray
DEL	Discoid lupus erythematosus
DGI	Disseminated gonococcal infection
ECG	Electrocardiogram
ITP	Idiopathic thrombocytopenic purpura
LBBB	Left bundle branch block
LDH	Lactate dehydrogenase
MCHC	Mean corpuscular hemoglobin concentration
MCV	Mean corpuscular volume
MR	Magnetic resonance
PCP	*Pneumocystis carinii* pneumonia
PML	Progressive multifocal leukoencephalopathy
PTCA	Percutaneous transluminal coronary angioplasty
RA	Rheumatoid arthritis
RBBB	Right bundle branch block
RF	Rheumatoid factor
RMSF	Rocky mountain spotted fever
SCLE	Subacute cutaneous lupus erythematosus

SLE	Systemic lupus erythematosus
SSc	Systemic sclerosis
TB	Tuberculosis
US	Ultrasonography
VPCs	Ventricular premature complexes
WBC	White blood cell
VF	Ventricular fibrillation

Pneumology

Sentences:

- Two measurements of lung volume can be used for respiratory diagnosis: RV and TLC.
- Thoracotomy is used to biopsy lesions that are too deep to vital structures for removal by VATS.
- HP is a term used for extrinsic allergic alveolitis.
- Life span for both female and male CF patients is similar (more or less 28 years)
- The ILDs are not caused by any defined infectious agents.
- About half of the patients with DVT have PTE.
- The narrowing of the upper airways during sleep predisposes to OSA.
- ARDS is characterized by increased permeability of the alveolar capillary barrier.

Definitions:

ARDs	Acute respiratory distress syndrome
CF	Cystic fibrosis
DVT	Deep venous thrombosis
HP	Hypersensitivity pneumonitis
ILDs	Interstitial lung disease
OSA	Obstructive sleep apnea
PTE	Pulmonary thromboembolism
RV	Residual volume
TLC	Total lung capacity
VATS	Video-assisted thoracic surgery

Nephrology

Sentences:

- The causes of ARF, RPRF, and CRF, although affecting the same organ, are different.
- ATN is typically induced by ischemia or nephrotoxins.

- The classic pathologic correlate of RPGN is crescent formation involving most glomeruli.
- Other glomerulopathies are MPGN, MCD and FSGS.
- Pathogenesis of RVT is not always clear, and its clinical manifestations depend on the severity of its occurrence.
- Renal failure is common in HUS and TTP.
- There are multiple forms of RTA, a disorder of renal acidification.

Definitions:

ARF	Acute renal failure
ATN	Acute tubular necrosis
CRF	Chronic renal failure
FSGS	Focal and segmental glomerulosclerosis
HUS	Hemolytic uremic syndrome
MCD	Minimal change disease
MPGN	Membranoproliferative glomerulopathies
RPGN	Rapidly progressive glomerulonephritis
RPRF	Rapidly progressive renal failure
RTA	Renal tubular acidosis
RVT	Renal vein thrombosis
TTP	Thrombotic thrombocytopenic purpura

Gastroenterology

Sentences:

- Ulcers can be more accurately detected using EDG rather than using GI X-ray examination.
- GU and DU are the major forms of peptic ulcer; these two terms include ulcers caused by NSAIDs and the ZES.
- 5% of patients with CD or UC (the major groups of chronic IBD) will have one or more relatives affected.
- One of the methods to reduce the pressure in the portal venous system in cirrhotic patients is the TIPS.

Definitions:

CD	Crohn disease
DU	Duodenal ulcer
EGD	Esophagogastroduodenoscopy
GI	Gastrointestinal
GU	Gastric ulcer
IBD	Inflammatory bowel disease
NSAIDs	Nonsteroidal anti-inflammatory drugs
TIPS	Transjugular intrahepatic portosystemic shunt

| UC | Ulcerative colitis |
| ZES | Zollinger-Ellison syndrome |

Abbreviation Lists

Although you should make your own abbreviation lists, we have created several classified by specialty. To begin with, check whether your own specialty's list is included; if not, start writing your own. Be patient ... this task can last the rest of your professional life.

General List

5FU	5-Fluorouracil
$a1$AT	$a1$-Antitrypsin
ABPA	Allergic bronchopulmonary aspergillosis
ACE	Angiotensin-converting enzyme
aCL	Antibodies to cardiolipin
ACTH	Adrenocorticotropic hormone
ADH	Antidiuretic hormone
ADPKD	Autosomal dominant polycystic kidney disease
AF	Atrial fibrillation
AFP	Alpha fetoprotein
AJCC	American Joint Cancer Commission
ALT	Alanine aminotransferase
AML	Acute myeloid leukemia
ANA	Antinuclear antibodies
APCs	Atrial premature complexes
APUD	Amine precursor uptake and decarboxylation system
ARDS	Acute respiratory distress syndrome
ARF	Acute renal failure
AS	Ankylosing spondylitis
AST	Aspartate aminotransferase
ATN	Acute tubular necrosis
AVP	Arginine vasopressin
BAL	Bronchoalveolar lavage
BCC	Basal cell carcinoma
BCG	Bacillus Calmette-Guérin
BMT	Bone marrow transplant
BP	Bullous pemphigoid
BPF	Brazilian purpuric fever
CBD	Common bile duct
CCK	Cholecystokinin
CD	Crohn disease

CEA	Carcinoembryonic antigen
CF	Cystic fibrosis
CML	Chronic myeloid leukemia
CMML	Chronic myelomonocytic leukemia
COPD	Chronic obstructive pulmonary disease
CP	Cicatricial pemphigoid
CRF	Chronic renal failure
CRH	Corticotropin-releasing hormone
CSF	Colony stimulating factor
CT	Computed tomography
CTX	Cholera toxin
CUPS	Cancer of unknown primary site
CWP	Coal workers' pneumoconiosis
CXR	Chest X-ray
DCIS	Ductal carcinoma in situ
DEL	Discoid lupus erythematosus
DGI	Disseminated gonococcal infection
DH	Dermatitis herpetiformis
DISH	Diffuse idiopathic skeletal hyperostosis
DRA	Dialysis-related amyloidosis
DRE	Digital rectal examination
DU	Duodenal ulcer
DVT	Deep venous thrombosis
EBA	Epidermolysis bullosa acquisita
EBV	Epstein Barr virus
ECG	Electrocardiogram
EGD	Esophagogastroduodenoscopy
ERCP	Endoscopic retrograde cholangiopancreatography
ESRD	End-stage renal disease
FAP	Familial amyloid polyneuropathies
FEV_1	Forced expiratory volume in 1 second
FMF	Familial Mediterranean fever
FSGS	Focal and segmental glomerulosclerosis
FSH	Follicle-stimulating hormone
GBM	Glomerular basement membrane
GCT	Germ cell tumor
GFR	Glomerular filtration rate
GGT	γ-Glutamyltranspeptidase, γ-Glutamyltranspherase
GH	Growth hormone
GHRH	Growth hormone-releasing hormone
GI	Gastrointestinal
GIP	Gastrin inhibitory peptide
GU	Gastric ulcer
HBV	Hepatitis B virus
hCG	Human chorionic gonadotropin
HCV	Hepatitis C virus

HIVAN	Human immunodeficiency virus-associated nephropathy
HOA	Hypertrophic osteoarthropathy
HP	Hypersensitivity pneumonitis
HPV	Human papilloma virus
HRT	Hormone replacement therapy
HSC	Hematopoietic stem cell
HUS	Hemolytic uremic syndrome
IBD	Inflammatory bowel disease
IBS	Irritable bowel syndrome
IL	Interleukin
ILD	Interstitial lung disease
IPSID	Immunoproliferative small intestinal disease (Mediterranean lymphoma)
ITP	Idiopathic thrombocytopenic purpura
JN	Juvenile nephronophthisis
LA	Lupus anticoagulant
LBBB	Left bundle branch block
LCDD	Light chain deposition disease
LDH	Lactate dehydrogenase
LES	Lower esophageal sphincter
LH	Luteinizing hormone
LIP	Lymphoid interstitial pneumonitis
MAC	*Mycobacterium avium* complex
MALT	Mucosa-associated lymphoid tissue
MCD	Medullary cystic disease
MCD	Minimal change disease
MCHC	Mean corpuscular hemoglobin concentration
MCTD	Mixed connective tissue disease
MCV	Mean corpuscular volume
MEN1	Type 1 multiple endocrine neoplasia
MPGN	Membranoproliferative glomerulopathies
MR	Magnetic resonance
MRI	Magnetic resonance imaging
NSAIDs	Nonsteroidal anti-inflammatory drugs
NUD	Non-ulcer dyspepsia
OA	Osteoarthritis
OCG	Oral cholecystography
ODTS	Organic dust toxic syndrome
OSA	Obstructive sleep apnea
PAH	Primary alveolar hypoventilation
PAN	Polyarteritis nodosa
PAP	Pulmonary alveolar proteinosis
PBC	Primary biliary cirrhosis
PCI	Prophylactic cranial irradiation
PCP	*Pneumocystis carinii* pneumonia
PEG	Percutaneous endoscopic gastrostomy

PF	Pemphigus foliaceus
PG	Pemphigoid gestationis
PIF	Prolactin inhibitory factor
PML	Progressive multifocal leukoencephalopathy
PNET	Peripheral primitive neuroectodermal tumor
PRA	Plasma renin activity
PRL	Prolactin
PSA	Prostate-specific antigen
PsA	Psoriatic arthritis
PTC	Percutaneous transhepatic cholangiography
PTE	Pulmonary thromboembolism
PTH	Parathyroid hormone
PV	Pemphigus vulgaris
RA	Rheumatoid arthritis
RBBB	Right bundle branch block
RBC	Red blood cell
RF	Rheumatoid factor
RMSF	Rocky mountain spotted fever
RPGN	Rapidly progressive glomerulonephritis
RPRF	Rapidly progressive renal failure
RTA	Renal tubular acidosis
RV	Residual volume
RVT	Renal vein thrombosis
SBC	Secondary biliary cirrhosis
SCC	Squamous cell carcinoma
SCID	Severe combined immunodeficiency
SCLE	Subacute cutaneous lupus erythematosus
SI	Serum iron
SIADH	Syndrome of inappropriate secretion of antidiuretic hormone
SLE	Systemic lupus erythematosus
SPB	Spontaneous bacterial peritonitis
SSc	Systemic sclerosis
SVCS	Superior vena cava syndrome
TB	Tuberculosis
TBB	Transbronchial biopsy
TGFβ	Transforming growth factor β
TIBC	Transferrin iron-binding capacity
TIPS	Transjugular intrahepatic portosystemic shunt
TLC	Total lung capacity
TNF	Tumor necrosis factor
TRH	Thyrotropin-releasing hormone
TSH	Thyroid-stimulating hormone
TTA	Transtracheal aspiration
TTP	Thrombotic thrombocytopenic purpura
UC	Ulcerative colitis

US	Ultrasonography
VATS	Video-assisted thoracic surgery
VC	Vital capacity
VF	Ventricular fibrillation
VIP	Vasoactive intestinal peptide
VPCs	Ventricular premature complexes
WBC	White blood cell
WDHA syndrome	Watery diarrhea, hypokalemia and achlorhydria syndrome (Verner-Morrison)
ZES	Zollinger-Ellison syndrome

Lists by Specialty

Anatomy

ACL	Anterior cruciate ligament of the knee
CBD	Common bile duct
CN	Cranial nerve
CNS	Central nervous system
DRUJ	Distal radioulnar joint
ECU	Extensor carpi ulnaris
ITB	Iliotibial band
IVC	Inferior vena cava
LCL	Lateral collateral ligament (knee, elbow)
MCL	Medial collateral ligament (knee, elbow)
MCP	Metacarpophalangeal
MTP	Metatarsophalangeal
NA	Nomina anatomica
PCL	Posterior cruciate ligament of the knee
RAS	Reticular activating system
RCL	Radial collateral ligament complex of the elbow
RDPA	Right descending pulmonary artery
SCM	Sternocleidomastoid muscle
ST	Scapulothoracic
TFCC	Triangular fibrocartilage complex
TMJ	Temporomandibular joint
TMT	Tarsometatarsal
UCL	Ulnar collateral ligament of the elbow
UPJ	Ureteropelvic junction

Biochemistry and Genetics

5-HT	5-Hydroxytryptamine
AA, aa	Amino acid
ACH, Ach	Acetylcholine
ACP	Acyl carrier protein
Ado	Adenosine
ADP	Adenosine 5c-diphosphate
ALA	Aminolevulinic acid
AMP	Adenosine monophosphate
ATP	Adenosine 5c-triphosphate
ATPase	Adenosine triphosphatase
CoA	Coenzyme A
DM	Dopamine
DNA	Deoxyribonucleic acid
GABA	γ-Aminobutyric acid
LT	Leukotrienes
NAD	Nicotinamide adenine dinucleotide
PABA	p-Aminobenzoic acid
PBG	Porphobilinogen
PCR	Polymerase chain reaction
PK	Pyruvate kinase
PP	Pyrophosphate
PRPP	5-Phospho-D-ribosyl 1-pyrophosphate
RIP	Radioimmunoprecipitation
RIST	Radioimmunosorbent test
RNA	Ribonucleic acid
RNP	Ribonucleoprotein
RT-PCR	Reverse transcriptase polymerase chain reaction
UDP	Uridine 5c-diphosphate

Cardiology, Cardiac and Vascular Surgery

AAA	Abdominal aortic aneurysm
AF	Atrial fibrillation
AFORMED phenomenon	Alternating failure of response, mechanical, to electrical depolarization of the heart
AH interval	Atrium–His interval
ALS	Advanced life support
AMI	Acute myocardial infarction
AN interval	Atrial deflection and the nodal potential
APSAC	Anisolated plasminogen streptokinase activator complex, for myocardial infarction
AR	Aortic regurgitation
AS	Aortic stenosis

A-V	Arteriovenous
AV	Atrioventricular
AVM	Arteriovenous malformation
aVF, aVL, aVR	Augmented electrocardiographic leads from the left foot, left arm, and right arm, respectively
CABG	Coronary artery bypass grafting
CAD	Coronary artery disease
CK	Creatine kinase
CK-MM, CK-BB, CK-MB	Creatine kinase isoenzymes
CPK	Creatine phosphokinase
CPR	Cardiopulmonary resuscitation
cTnT	Cardiac-specific troponin T, in myocardial infarction
CVP	Central venous pressure
DA	Ductus arteriosus
ECMO	Extracorporeal-membrane oxygenation
ECG	Electrocardiogram
EKG	Electrocardiogram
HOMC	Hypertrophic obstructive cardiomyopathy
HV	His-ventricular conduction time
ICD	Implantable cardioverter-defibrillator
LVET	Left ventricular ejection time
LVOT	Left ventricle outflow tract
MASS	Mitral valve prolapse, aortic anomalies, skeletal changes, and skin changes
MAT	Multifocal atrial tachycardia
MI	Myocardial infarction
MR	Mitral regurgitation
MS	Mitral stenosis
MVP	Mitral valve prolapse
PAPVR	Partial anomalous pulmonary venous return
PCWP	Pulmonary capillary wedge pressure
PEA	Pulseless electrical activity
PPPPPP	Pain, pallor, paresthesia, pulselessness, paralysis, prostration (the symptom complex of acute arterial occlusion)
PTCA	Percutaneous transluminal coronary angioplasty
RVOT	Right ventricle outflow tract
S-A	Sinuatrial
TAPVC	Total anomalous pulmonary venous connection
TED	Thromboembolic disease
WPW	Wolff-Parkinson-White disease

Clinical History

AC, a.c.	*Ante cibum* (before a meal)
ADR	Adverse drug reaction
AVPU	Alert, responsive to verbal stimuli, responsive to painful stimuli, and unresponsive (assessment of mental status)
BID, b.i.d.	*Bis in die* (twice a day)
BP	Blood pressure
CC	Chief complaint
DM	Diastolic murmur
DNR	Do not resuscitate
DOA	Dead on arrival
DRE	Digital rectal examination
DTR	Deep tendon reflex
IV, i.v.	Intravenous
LUQ	Left upper quadrant (of abdomen)
NPO	*Nil per os* (nothing by mouth)
OD	Overdose
PCA	Patient-controlled analgesia
PO	*Per os* (by mouth, oral)
POMR	Problem-oriented medical record
ppm	Parts per million
PRE	Progressive-resistance exercise
p.r.n.	*Pro re nata* (according to circumstances, may require)
PT	Physical therapy/therapist
RDA	Recommended daily allowance
RLL	Right lower lobe (of lung)
RLQ	Right lower quadrant (of abdomen)
RML	Right middle lobe (of lung)
RUL	Right upper lobe (of lung)
RUQ	Right upper quadrant (of abdomen)
SM	Systolic murmur
SOAP	Subjective, objective, assessment, and plan (used in problem-oriented records)
SQ	Subcutaneous
TPN	Total parenteral nutrition
VR	Vocal resonance

Dentistry

DEJ	Dentinoenamel junction
DMF	Decayed, missing, and filled (permanent teeth caries index)
DMFS	Decayed, filled, or missing tooth surfaces
DMFT	Decayed, missing, or filled teeth

FDI	Fédération Dentaire Internationale; a system of identifying
nomenclature	teeth
GPI	Gingival-periodontal index
PI	Periodontal index

Dermatology

BCC	Basal cell carcinoma
BP	Bullous pemphigoid
CP	Cicatricial pemphigoid
DEL	Discoid lupus erythematosus
DH	Dermatitis herpetiformis
EBA	Epidermolysis bullosa acquisita
PF	Pemphigus foliaceus
PG	Pemphigoid gestationis
PsA	Psoriatic arthritis
PTK	Phototherapeutic keratectomy
PUPPP	Pruritic urticarial papules and plaques of pregnancy
PUVA	Psoralen plus ultraviolet A irradiation
PV	Pemphigus vulgaris
SCLE	Subacute cutaneous lupus erythematosus
TAD	Transient acantholytic dermatosis
TEN	Toxic epidermal necrolysis

Endocrinology and Metabolism

AASH	Adrenal androgen-stimulating hormone
ABP	Androgen binding protein
ACE	Angiotensin-converting enzyme
ACTH	Adrenocorticotropic hormone
ADH	Antidiuretic hormone
ANP	Atrial natriuretic peptide
APECED	Autoimmune polyendocrinopathy-candidiasis-ectodermal dystrophy
APUD	Amine precursor uptake and decarboxylation
AS	Alport syndrome
AVP	Arginine vasopressin
BMI	Body mass index
BMR	Basal metabolic rate
BSA	Body surface area
CCK	Cholecystokinin
CDs	Chondrodysplasias
CRF	Corticotropin-releasing factor
CRH	Corticotropin-releasing hormone
DHEA	Dehydroepiandrosterone
DKA	Diabetic ketoacidosis

DM	Diabetes mellitus
EB	Epidermolysis bullosa
EDS	Ehlers-Danlos syndrome
FCHL	Familial combined hyperlipidemia
FFM	Fat-free body mass
FHH	Familial hypocalciuric hypercalcemia
FRC	Functional residual capacity
FSH	Follicle-stimulating hormone
GH	Growth hormone
GHRH	Growth hormone-releasing hormone
GnRH	Gonadotropin-releasing hormone
GTHR	Generalized thyroid hormone resistance
HAIR-AN syndrome	Hyperandrogenism, insulin resistance, and acanthosis nigricans syndrome
HCP	Hereditary coproporphyria
HCS	Human chorionic somatomammotropic hormone
HEP	Hepatoerythropoietic porphyria
HVA	Homovanillic acid
IAP	Intermittent acute porphyria
IDDM	Insulin-dependent diabetes mellitus
IGF	Insulin-like growth factor
IUD	Intrauterine device
IVF	In vitro fertilization
LATS	Long-acting thyroid stimulator
LCAT	Lecithin cholesterol acyltransferase
LH	Luteinizing hormone
MEN	Multiple endocrine neoplasia
MRF	Melanotropin-releasing factor
MS	Marfan syndrome
MTC	Medullary thyroid carcinoma
NIDDM	Non-insulin-dependent diabetes mellitus
NPD	Niemann-Pick disease
OBLA	Onset of blood lactate accumulation
OI	Osteogenesis imperfecta
PCT	Porphyria cutanea tarda
PHP	Panhypopituitarism
PIF	Prolactin inhibitory factor
PKU	Phenylketonuria
POCD	Polycystic ovary disease
POMC	Pro-opiomelanocortin
PRA	Plasma renin activity
PRF	Prolactin-releasing factor
PRL	Prolactin
PTH	Parathyroid hormone
SES	Sick euthyroid syndrome
SIADH	Syndrome of inappropriate antidiuretic hormone

SIH	Somatotropin release-inhibiting hormone
SRH	Somatotropin-releasing hormone
TRH	Thyrotropin-releasing hormone
TSH	Thyroid-stimulating hormone
TSI	Thyroid-stimulating immunoglobulins
VIP	Vasoactive intestinal polypeptide
VP	Variegate porphyria
XLSA	X-linked sideroblastic anemia

Gastroenterology

APC	Adenomatous polyposis coli
CD	Crohn disease
DU	Duodenal ulcus
GI	Gastrointestinal
LES	Lower esophageal sphincter
LFT	Liver function test
ERCP	Endoscopic retrograde cholangiopancreatography
ERS	Endoscopic retrograde sphincterotomy
FEES	Fiberoptic endoscopic examination of swallowing
GERD	Gastroesophageal reflux disease

General Surgery

D&C	Dilation and curettage
D&E	Dilation and evacuation
LEEP	Loop electrocautery excision procedure
TEP	Tracheoesophageal puncture

Health Policy, Health Institutions

ABN	Advance beneficiary notice
ADA	Americans with Disabilities Act
ALD	Assistive listening device
ANSI	American National Standards Institute
CDC	Centers for Disease Control and Prevention; previously known as the Communicable Disease Center
DALYs	Disability-adjusted life years
FDA	Food and Drug Administration of the United States Department of Health and Human Services
HCFA	Health Care Financing Administration
HRSA	Health Resources and Services Administration
ICD	International Classification of Diseases
NIH	National Institutes of Health (US Public Health Service)
PRN	Peer-review organization
QC	Quality control
USPHS	United States Public Health Service

Hematology and Immunology

AC	Anticoagulant
ACT	Activated clotting time
Ag	Antigen
ADH	Alcohol dehydrogenase
AHF	Antihemophilic factor A
ALL	Acute lymphocytic leukemia
ALT	Alanine aminotransferase
AP	Alkaline phosphatase
APTT	Activated partial thromboplastin time
AST	Aspartate aminotransferase
ATL	Adult T-cell leukemia
ATL	Adult T-cell lymphoma
BUN	Blood urea nitrogen
CBC	Complete blood count
CD	Cluster of differentiation
CGD	Chronic granulomatous disease
CGL	Chronic granulocytic leukemia
CML	Chronic myelocytic leukemia
CRP	C-reactive protein
DIC	Disseminated intravascular coagulation
ESR	Erythrocyte sedimentation rate
FAB	French-American-British classification system
FEL	Familial erythrophagocytic lymphohistiocytosis
FMLH	Familial hemophagocytic lymphohistiocytosis
G-CSF	Granulocyte colony-stimulating factor
GOT	Glutamic-oxaloacetic transaminase
GPT	Glutamic-pyruvic transaminase
GVHR	Graft versus host reaction
Hb	Hemoglobin
Hct	Hematocrit
HDL	High-density lipoprotein
HGF	Hematopoietic growth factor
HLA	Human leukocyte antigen (major histocompatibility complex in humans)
HMWK	High molecular weight kininogen
IgA, IgD, IgE, IgG, IgM	Immunoglobulins
IFN	Interferon
IL	Interleukin
INR	International normalized ratio
ITP	Idiopathic thrombocytopenic purpura
LAD	Leukocyte adhesion deficiency
LDH	Lactate dehydrogenase
LDL	Low-density lipoprotein

LET	Leukocyte esterase test
MCH	Mean corpuscular hemoglobin
MCHC	Mean corpuscular hemoglobin concentration
MCV	Mean corpuscular volume
MGUS	Monoclonal gammapathy of unknown significance
MHC	Major histocompatibility complex
NK cells	Natural killer cells
PCH	Paroxysmal cold hemoglobinuria
PDLL	Poorly differentiated lymphocytic lymphoma
PNH	Paroxysmal nocturnal hemoglobinuria
PNP	Platelet neutralization procedure
PPCA	Proserum prothrombin conversion accelerator
PT	Prothrombin time
PTA	Plasma thromboplastin antecedent
PTT	Partial thromboplastin time
rbc	Red blood cell
RBC	Red-cell blood count
REAL	Revised European-American classification of lymphoid neoplasms
SPCA	Serum prothrombin conversion accelerator
TIBC	Total iron binding capacity
VHDL	Very high density lipoprotein
VLDL	Very low density lipoprotein
VMA	Vanillylmandelic acid
WBC	White-cell blood count

The Hospital

CCU	Coronary care unit
CCU	Critical care unit
ECU	Emergency care unit
EMS	Emergency medical service
ER	Emergency room
ICF	Intermediate care facility
ICU	Intensive care unit

Infectious Diseases

AIDS	Acquired immunodeficiency syndrome
CSD	Catscratch disease
FIA	Feline infectious anemia
HIV-1	Human immunodeficiency virus-1
MOTT	Mycobacteria other than *Mycobacterium tuberculosis* complex
PMC	Pseudomembranous colitis
PML	Progressive multifocal leukoencephalopathy

SBE	Subacute bacterial endocarditis
STD	Sexually transmitted disease
STORCH	Syphilis, toxoplasmosis, other infections, rubella, cytomegalovirus infection, and herpes simplex (fetal infections that can cause congenital malformations)
TB	Tuberculosis
TORCH syndrome	Toxoplasmosis, other infections, rubella, cytomegalovirus infection, and herpes simplex
TSS	Toxic shock syndrome
UTI	Urinary tract infection

Internal Medicine

ACLA	Anticardiolipin lupus anticoagulant
ADL	Activities of daily living
ANA	Antinuclear antibody
ANCA	Antineutrophil cytoplasmic antibody
ANF	Antinuclear factor
APS	Antiphospholipid antibody syndrome
AS	Ankylosing spondylitis
CREST	Calcinosis, Raynaud's phenomenon, esophageal motility disorders, sclerodactyly, and telangiectasia
DLE	Discoid lupus erythematosus
DVT	Deep venous thrombosis
EP	Endogenous pyrogen
FUO	Fever of unknown origin
HHIE-S	Hearing handicap inventory for the elderly
IM	Internal medicine
LE	Lupus erythematosus
PUO	Pyrexia of unknown (or undetermined) origin
RA	Rheumatoid arthritis
SLE	Systemic lupus erythematosus

Microbiology

AFA fixative	Alcohol, formalin, and acetic acid used for the fixation of certain parasites
AFB	Acid-fast bacillus
ASO	Anti-streptolysin O
BCG	Bacillus Calmette-Guérin
CFU	Colony-forming unit
CMV	Cytomegalovirus
DPT	Diphtheria-pertussis-tetanus (vaccine)
DTaP	Diphtheria, tetanus, and acellular pertussis vaccine
EBV	Epstein-Barr virus
EHEC	Enterohemorrhagic *Escherichia coli*

ELISA	Enzyme-linked immunosorbent assay
EPEC	Enteropathogenic *Escherichia coli*
FTA-ABS	Fluorescent treponemal antibody absorption
GLC	Gas-liquid chromatography
HACEK group	A group of Gram-negative bacteria (*Haemophilus* spp., *Actinobacillus actinomycetemcomitans, Cardiobacterium hominis, Eikenella corrodens, Kingella kingae*)
HBcAg	Hepatitis B core antigen
HBeAg	Hepatitis B e antigen
HBIG	Hepatitis B immune globulin
HBsAg	Hepatitis B surface antigen
HBV	Hepatitis B virus
HCV	Hepatitis C virus
HDV	Hepatitis D virus
HEV	Hepatitis E virus
HGV	Hepatitis G virus
HPV	Human papilloma virus
HSV	Herpes simplex virus
HTLV-III	Human T-cell lymphotropic virus type III (HIV-I virus)
LAV	Lymphadenopathy-associated virus
MAI	*Mycobacterium avium-intracellulare*
MID	Minimal infecting dose
PPLO	Pleuropneumonia-like organisms
SK	Streptokinase
TNTC	Too numerous to count (usually cells in a urine specimen)
VDRL	Venereal Disease Research Laboratories
VZV	Varicella-zoster virus

Nephrology

ADPKD	Autosomal dominant polycystic kidney disease
ALG	Antilymphocyte globulin in renal transplantation
ANA	Antinuclear antibody
ANCA	Antineutrophil cytoplasmic antibodies
ARF	Acute renal failure
ASO	Antistreptolysin O antibody titer
ATN	Acute tubular necrosis
BUN	Blood urea nitrogen
CAPD	Continuous ambulatory peritoneal dialysis
CAVHD	Continuous arteriovenous hemodiafiltration
CCPD	Continuous cyclic peritoneal dialysis
CRF	Chronic renal failure
CVVHD	Continuous venovenous hemodiafiltration
DRA	Dialysis-related amyloidosis
EMC	Essential mixed cryoglobulinemia

ERBF	Effective renal blood flow
ERPF	Effective renal plasma flow
ERT	Estrogen replacement therapy
ESRD	End-stage renal disease
FF	Filtration fraction
FSGS	Focal and segmental glomerulosclerosis
GBM	Glomerular basement membrane
GFR	Glomerular filtration rate
GN	Glomerulonephritis
HIVAN	Human immunodeficiency virus-associated nephropathy
HSP	Henoch-Schönlein purpura
HUS	Hemolytic-uremic syndrome
IPD	Intermittent peritoneal dialysis
IVP	Intravenous pyelogram
JN	Juvenile nephronophthisis
LCDD	Light chain deposition disease
MCD	Medullary cystic disease
MDRD	Modification of diet in renal disease
MPGN	Membranoproliferative glomerulonephritis
MSK	Medullary sponge kidney
NDI	Nephrogenic diabetes insipidus
NSAID	Nonsteroidal antiinflammatory drug
PRA	Plasma renin activity
RBF	Renal blood flow
RPF	Renal plasma flow
RPGN	Rapidly progressive glomerulonephritis
RPRF	Rapidly progressive renal failure
RTA	Renal tubular acidosis
RVT	Renal vein thrombosis
TBM	Thin basement membrane disease
URR	Urea reduction ratio

Neurology

AD	Alzheimer disease
ADEM	Acute disseminated encepahalomyelitis
ADNFLE	Nocturnal frontal lobe epilepsy
AGM	Awakening grand mal
AHL	Acute hemorrhagic leukoencephalitis
ALS	Amyotrophic lateral sclerosis
ANS	Autonomic nervous system
AVED	Ataxia with vitamin E deficiency
AVM	Arteriovenous malformation
BAEP	Brainstem auditory evoked potential
BBB	Blood-brain barrier
BMD	Becker muscular dystrophy

BSE	Bovine spongiform encephalopathy
CADASIL	Cerebellar autosomal dominant arteriopathy with subcortical infarcts
CCD	Central cord disease
CIPD	Chronic inflammatory demyelinating polyneuropathy
CJD	Creutzfeldt-Jakob disease
CNS	Central nervous system
CSF	Cerebrospinal fluid
CSFP	Cerebrospinal fluid pressure
CVA	Cerebrovascular accident
DMD	Duchenne muscular dystrophy
DOMS	Delayed onset muscle soreness
ECS	Electrocerebral silence
EEG	Electroencephalogram
EMG	Electromyogram
ENG	Electronystagmography
EPMR	Epilepsy progressive with mental retardation
EP	Evoked potential
FAP	Familial amyloid polyneuropathy
FSP	Familial spastic paraplegia
GABA	γ-Aminobutyric acid
GBS	Guillain-Barré syndrome
HD	Huntington disease
ICP	Intracranial pressure
ILAE	International league against epilepsy
INO	Internuclear ophthalmoplegia
JME	Juvenile myoclonic epilepsy
LEMS	Lambert-Eaton myasthenic syndrome
LTM	Long-term memory
MAOS	Monoamine oxidase inhibitors
MD	Muscular dystrophy
ME	Myalgic encephalomyelitis
MELAS	Mitochondrial myopathy, encephalopathy, lactic acidosis, and stroke-like episodes (one of the mitochondrial disorders)
MERRF	Myoclonic epilepsy with ragged red fiber myopathy (one of the mitochondrial disorders)
MG	Myasthenia gravis
MJD	Machado-Joseph disease
MS	Multiple sclerosis
MSA	Multiple system atrophy
NARP	Neuropathy, ataxia, retinitis pigmentosa syndrome (one of the inherited mitochondrial disorders)
NPH	Normal-pressure hydrocephalus
NREM	Non-rapid eye movement
OBS	Organic brain syndrome

PLS	Primary lateral sclerosis
PROMM	Proximal myotonic myopathy
PTSD	Posttraumatic stress disorder
PVS	Persistent vegetative state
REM	Rapid eye movements
SAH	Subarachnoid hemorrhage
SCA	Spinocerebellar ataxia
SCCD	Subacute cortical cerebellar degeneration
SEP	Somatosensory evoked potential
SER	Somatosensory evoked response
SSPE	Subacute sclerosing panencephalitis
SSRI	Selective serotonin reuptake inhibitor
TCA	Tricyclic antidepressant
TIA	Transient ischemic attack
TMB	Transient monocular blindness
VEP	Visual evoked potential

Obstetrics and Gynecology

AFP	a-Fetoprotein
AID	Artificial insemination donor
AIH	Artificial insemination (homologous)
CIN	Cervical intraepithelial neoplasia
CHL	Crown-heel length
CRL	Crown-rump length
DES	Diethylstilbestrol
GIFT	Gamete intrafallopian transfer
HCG	Human chorionic gonadotropin
HRT	Hormone replacement therapy
IUCD, IUD	Intrauterine contraceptive device
IUI	Intrauterine insemination
LFT	Left frontotransverse position
LMA	Left mentoanterior position
LMP	Left mentoposterior position
LMT	Left mentotransverse position
LOT	Left occipitotransverse position
LSA	Left sacroanterior position
LSP	Left sacroposterior position
LST	Left sacrotransverse position
MP	Mentoposterior position
MPC	Mucopurulent cervicitis
OA	Occipitoanterior position
OB/GYN	Obstetrics and gynecology
PID	Pelvic inflammatory disease
PMS	Premenstrual syndrome
RFP	Right frontoposterior position

RFT	Right frontotransverse position
RMA	Right mentoanterior position
RMP	Right mentoposterior position
RMT	Right mentotransverse position
ROA	Right occipitoanterior position
ROP	Right occipitoposterior position
ROT	Right occipitotransverse position
RPO	Right posterior oblique (a radiographic position)
RSA	Right sacroanterior position
RSP	Right sacroposterior position
RST	Right sacrotransverse position
SP	Sacroposterior position
VACTERL syndrome	Abnormalities of vertebrae, anus, cardiovascular tree, trachea, esophagus, renal system, and limb buds (associated with administration of sex steroids during early pregnancy)

Oncology

AGCUS	Atypical glandular cells of undetermined significance
ASCUS	Atypical squamous cells of undetermined significance
CEA	Carcinoembryonic antigen
CIS	Carcinoma in situ
CMV	Cisplatin, methotrexate, and vinblastine (a cancer drug combination treatment)
CUPS	Cancer of unknown primary site
HGSIL	High-grade squamous intraepithelial lesion
LGSIL	Low-grade squamous intraepithelial lesion
MFH	Malignant fibrous hystiocytoma
PNET	Primitive neuroectodermal tumors
TAF	Tumor angiogenic factor
TNM	staging Tumor-node-metastasis

Ophthalmology

AC/A	Accommodative convergence – accommodation ratio
ARN	Acute retinal necrosis
DCG	Dacryocystography
DUSN	Diffuse unilateral subacute neuroretinitis
EOG	Electrooculography
ERG	Electroretinogram
LE	Left eye
PORN	Progressive outer retinal necrosis
RE	Right eye
TRIC	Trachoma and inclusion conjunctivitis

Orthopedics

ABC	Aneurysmal bone cyst
A-E	Above-the-elbow (amputation)
A-K	Above-the-knee (amputation)
ALPSA	Anterior labroligamentous periosteal sleeve avulsion
B-E	Below-the-elbow (amputation)
BHAGL	Bony humeral avulsion of glenohumeral ligament
B-K	Below-the-knee (amputation)
CPPD	Calcium pyrophosphate dihydrate deposition
CTD	Cumulative trauma disorders
DISH	Diffuse idiopathic skeletal hyperostosis
DISI	Dorsal intercalated segmental instability
EDM	Multiple epiphyseal dysplasia
GLAD	Glenolabral articular disruption
HAGL	Humeral avulsion of glenohumeral ligament
HNP	Herniated nucleus pulposus
HOA	Hypertrophic osteoarthropathy
ITOH	Idiopathic transient osteoporosis of the hip
MAST	Military antishock trousers
OCD	Osteochondritis dissecans
OI	Osteogenesis imperfecta
OSMED	Otospondylomegaepiphyseal dysplasia
PVNS	Pigmented villonodular synovitis
RSD	Reflex sympathetic dystrophy
SAPHO syndrome	Synovitis, acne, pustulosis, hyperostosis, and osteitis
SCFE	Slipped capital femoral epiphysis
SEDC	Spondyloepiphyseal dysplasia congenita
SLAC	Scapholunate advanced collapse
SLAP	Superior labrum, anterior-posterior (lesion of the glenoid labrum)
TMJ	Temporomandibular joint
TOS	Thoracic outlet syndrome

Otorhinolaryngology

ABG	Air-bone gap in otoscopy (conductive hearing loss)
ABR	Auditory brainstem response
ART	Acoustic reflex threshold
BSER	Brainstem evoked response
CIC	Completely in the canal hearing aid
ENT	Ears, nose, and throat
NUG	Necrotizing ulcerative gingivitis
OAE	Otoacoustic emission

| SISI | Small increment sensitivity index (test for cochlear damage) |

Pediatrics

BIDS	Brittle hair, impaired intelligence, decreased fertility, and short stature
CDH	Congenital dislocation of the hip
DDH	Developmental dysplasia of hip
LEOPARD syndrome	Lentigines, electrocardiographic abnormalities, ocular hypertelorism, pulmonary stenosis, abnormalities of genitalia, retardation of growth, and deafness
SBS	Shaken baby syndrome
SIDS	Sudden infant death syndrome

Pharmacology

ACEI	Angiotensin-converting enzyme inhibitor
AZT	Azidothymidine
CDCA	Chenodeoxycholic acid
DMARD	Disease-modifying antirheumatic drugs
MAOI	Monoamine oxidase inhibitors
MPD	Maximum permissible dose
MRD, mrd	Minimal reacting dose
MS	Morphine sulfate
NSAID	Nonsteroidal anti-inflammatory drug
SSRI	Selective serotonin reuptake inhibitor

Pneumology

$A\text{-}aO_2$ difference	Alveolar-arterial oxygen partial pressure difference
ABG	Air-bone gap
ABG	Arterial blood gas
ABPA	Allergic bronchopulmonary aspergillosis
ACMV	Assist control mode ventilation
ALI	Acute lung injury
ARDS	Adult respiratory distress syndrome
ARF	Acute respiratory failure
Auto-PEEP	Auto-positive end-expiratory pressure
BAL	Bronchoalveolar lavage
BALT	Bronchus-associated lymphoid tissue
BiPAP	Bilevel positive airway pressure
BOOP	Bronchiolitis obliterans with organizing pneumonia
BPF	Bronchopleural fistula
BVM	Bag-valve-mask device

CF	Cystic fibrosis
CFTR	Cystic fibrosis transmembrane regulator
CO	Cardiac output
COPD	Chronic obstructive pulmonary disease
CPAP	Continuous positive airway pressure
CPPB	Continuous positive pressure breathing
CSA	Central sleep apnea
CWP	Coal workers' pneumoconiosis
DIC	Disseminated intravascular coagulation
DL_{CO}	Diffusing capacity of the lung for carbon monoxide
2,3-DPG	2,3-Diphosphoglycerate
DVT	Deep venous thrombosis
ECHO	Extracorporeal membrane oxygenation
ERV	Expiratory reserve volume
FEF	Forced expiratory flow
FEFn–n%	Forced expiratory flow between n% and n% of the vital capacity
FET	Forced expiratory time
FEV 1	Forced expiratory volume in 1 second
FIO_2	Fractional concentration of inspired O_2
FRC	Functional residual capacity
FVC	Forced vital capacity
HFV	High-frequency ventilation
HP	Hypersensitivity pneumonitis
HRCT	High-resolution CT
IC	Inspiratory capacity
ILD	Interstitial lung disease
IMV	Intermittent mandatory ventilation
IPC	Intermittent pneumatic compression
IPF	Idiopathic pulmonary fibrosis
IPPV	Intermittent positive pressure ventilation
IRV	Inspiratory reserve volume
MBC	Maximum breathing capacity
MEP	Maximum expiratory pressure
MIP	Maximum inspiratory pressure
MMFR	Maximal midexpiratory flow rate
MOF	Multiple organ failure
NEEP	Negative end-expiratory pressure
NO	Nitric oxide
ODTS	Organic dust toxic syndrome
OSA	Obstructive sleep apnea
PAH	Primary alveolar hypoventilation
PAP	Pulmonary alveolar proteinosis
PAP	Pulmonary arterial pressure
PAV	Proportional assist ventilation
PCV	Pulmonary vascular resistance

PCWP	Pulmonary capillary wedge pressure
PEEP	Positive end-expiratory pressure
PEFR	Peak flowmeter
PEFR	Peak expiratory flow rate
PF	Pleural fluid
PFT	Pulmonary function test
PIOPED	Prospective investigation of pulmonary embolism diagnosis
PMF	Progressive massive fibrosis
PNPB	Positive-negative pressure breathing
PPV	Positive pressure ventilation
PSB	Protected double-sheathed brush
PSV	Pressure-support ventilation
PTE	Pulmonary thromboembolism
Ptp	Transpulmonary pressure
PVR	Pulmonary vascular resistance
RQ	Respiratory quotient
RV	Residual volume
SIMV	Synchronized intermittent mandatory ventilation
TBB	Transbronchial biopsy
TLC	Total lung capacity
TTA	Transtracheal aspiration
VA	Alveolar ventilation
VATS	Video-assisted thoracic surgery
VC	Vital capacity
Vt	Tidal volume
VTE	Venous thromboembolism

Psychiatry

ADD	Attention deficit disorder
ADHD	Attention deficit hyperactivity disorder
CA	Chronological age
DSM-IV	Diagnostic and statistical manual (an American Psychiatric Association publication that classifies mental illnesses)
DT	Delirium tremens
ECT	Electroconvulsive therapy
IQ	Intelligence quotient
MA	Mental age
OCD	Obsessive compulsive disorder
SAD	Seasonal affective disorder
STM	Short-term memory

Radiology

DTPA	Diethylene triamine pentaacetic acid (a binding substance for both Gd and 99m-Tc)
ALARA	As low as reasonably achievable (radiation dosages)
AMBER	Advanced multiple-beam equalization radiography
BE	Barium enema
CT	Computed tomography
DICOM	Digital Imaging and Communications in Medicine (a joint standard of the American College of Radiology and National Equipment Manufacturers' Association)
DSA	Digital subtraction angiography
EBT	Electron beam tomography
FSE	Fast spin echo (a magnetic resonance sequence)
Fr	French scale (catheters)
GRASS	Gradient-recalled acquisition in the steady state (a magnetic resonance sequence)
GRE	Gradient echo imaging (a magnetic resonance sequence)
HRCT	High-resolution computed tomography
IVU	Intravenous urogram
LAO	Left anterior oblique position
LPO	Left posterior oblique position
MIP	Maximum intensity projection
MRI	Magnetic resonance imaging
PACS	Picture archive and communication system (a computer network for digitized radiological images and reports)
PET	Positron emission tomography
PTA	Percutaneous transluminal angioplasty
PTHC, PTC	Percutaneous transhepatic cholangiography
RAO	Right anterior oblique
SE	Spin echo (a magnetic resonance sequence)
SNR	Signal-to-noise ratio
SPECT	Single photon emission computed tomography
STIR	Short tau inversion recovery imaging (a magnetic resonance sequence)
TE	Echo time (in magnetic resonance spin echo pulse sequences)
TIPS	Transjugular intrahepatic portosystemic shunt
TR	Repetition time
UGI	Upper gastrointestinal series
VCUG	Voiding cystourethrogram
XR	X-ray

Urology

BPH	Benign prostatic hyperplasia
ESWL	Extracorporeal shock wave lithotripsy
GU	Genitourinary
PIN	Prostatic intraepithelial neoplasia
PSA	Prostate-specific antigen
SUI	Stress urinary incontinence

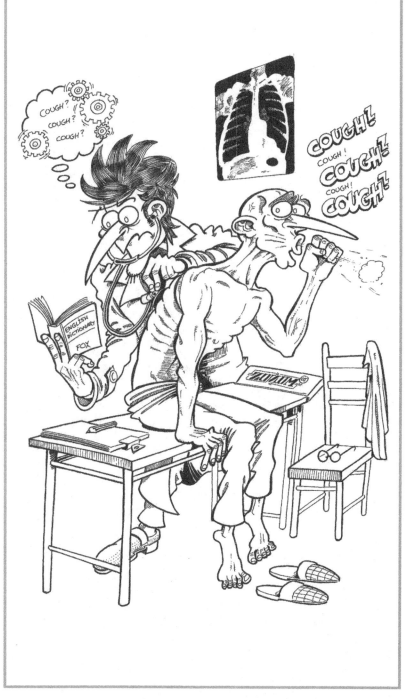

Unit VIII The Clinical History

Communication Skills

Good communication between doctor and patient is vital in order to establish an accurate medical history. In the following pages we show several key sentences which can help you when interviewing a patient.

1. Greeting and introducing oneself:
   - Good morning, Mr. Lee. Come and sit down. I'm Dr. Vida.
   - Good afternoon, Mrs. Lafontaine. Take a seat, please.

2. Invitation to describe symptoms:
   - Well now, what seems to be the problem?
   - Well, how can I help you?
   - Would you please tell me how I can help you?
   - Your GP (general practitioner) says you've been having trouble with your right shoulder. Tell me about it.
   - My colleague Dr. Sanders says your left knee has been aching lately. Is that correct?

3. Instructions for undressing:
   - Would you mind taking off all your clothes except your underwear? (men).
   - Would you please take off all your clothes except your underwear and bra? (women).
   - You should take off your underwear too.
   - Lie on the couch and cover yourself with the blanket.
   - Lie on the stretcher with your shoes and socks off, please.
   - Roll your sleeve up, please, I'm going to examine your elbow.

4. Instructions for position on couch:
   - Lie down, please (supine position).
   - Lie on your tummy, please (prone position).
   - Please turn over and lie on your back again.
   - Roll over onto your right side.
   - Sit up and bend you knees.
   - Lean forward.
   - Get off the stretcher.

- Stand up, please.
- Lie on your back with your knees bent and your legs wide apart.
- Lie on your tummy and relax.
- Let yourself go loose.

5. Instructions to get dressed:
   - You can get dressed now. Take your time, we are not in a hurry.
   - Please get dressed. Take your time, we are not in a hurry.

6. No treatment:
   - There is nothing wrong with you.
   - This will clear up on its own.
   - There doesn't seem to be anything wrong with your shoulder.

The Chart

A typical completed clinical history chart is shown in Table 1. As you can see, in case you were not aware of it, a chart is almost entirely written in doctors' shorthand. Get a chart, photocopy it and go over it thoroughly; the sooner you do it the better.

Taking a Clinical History

Since we take for granted that your English level allows you to understand most of the possible questions to ask patients and being aware that every specialty has questions of its own, this section does not intend to be an ordinary guide. Its only intention is to serve as an example and it is aimed at encouraging you to create your own list of questions and comments.

In Table 2 we provide a list of common phrases that patients use to describe their symptoms and the meaning of these phrases.

Questions and Commands

1. To begin the interview:
   - Well now, how can I help you?
   - What's brought you along today?
   - What can I do for you?
   - What seems to be the problem?
   - Well Mr. Goyen, what's the trouble?
   - Your doctor says you've been having trouble with your knees. Tell me about it.
   - How long has/have it/they been bothering you?

Table 1. Typical clinical history chart

Surname (1st):	Hall	Surname (2nd):	First name(s): Kevin
Age: 32	Sex: M		Marital status: M
Occupation:	Truck driver		
Present complaint:	Frontal headaches 3/12[a]. Worse in a.m. "Dull"[b], "throbbing"[c]. Relieved by lying down. Also c/o[d] progressive deafness.		
O/E[e]: General condition:	Obese, 1.65 m tall, 85 kg weight		
ENT[f]:	Wax[g] ++, both sides		
RS[h]:	NAD[i]		
CVS[j]:	P[k] 80/min reg[l], BP[m] 180/120, HS[n] Normal		
GIS[o]:			
GUS[p]:			
CNS[q]:	Fundi[r] normal		
Immediate past history: Weight gain			
Points of note:	None		
Investigations[s]: Urine -ve[t] for sugar and albumin Retinoscopy			
Diagnosis:	Hypertension		
Management:			
Date: 26/03/99		Signature: Peter Weiss MD.	

[a] *3/12* For 3 months (similarly, *6/52* 6 weeks and *4/7* 4 days).
[b] *Dull* "A dull sort of ache". Not felt distinctly. Not sharp.
[c] *Throbbing* Beating more rapidly than usual.
[d] *c/o* Complains of.
[e] *O/E* On examination.
[f] *ENT* Ear–nose–throat.
[g] *Wax* Wax within the external auditory canal.
[h] *RS* Respiratory system.
[i] *NAD* Nothing abnormal detected, also Non-apparent distress.
[j] *CVS* Cardiovascular system.
[k] *P* Pulse.
[l] *reg* Regular (other: SR Sinus rhythm).
[m] *BP* Blood pressure.
[n] *HS* Heart sounds.
[o] *GIS* Gastrointestial system.

continued fotenote to Table 1
^p *GUS* Genitourinary system.
^q *CNS* Central nervous system.
^r *Fundi* Equivalent to "found".
^s *Investigations* Tests.
^t *–ve* negative (*+ve* positive).

   - How long have you had it/them?
   - How long have you been ill?
   - Did it start all of a sudden?
   - How many days have you been indisposed?
   - What do you think the reason is?
   - Do you think there is any explanation?
2. General questions/commands:
   - How many times?
   - How much?
   - How often?
   - How old are you?
   - Have you had bleeding?
   - Have you had fever?
   - Have you had any nose bleeding?
   - Have you lost weight lately?
   - Open your mouth, please.
   - Please remove your clothing.
   - Raise your arm.
   - Raise it more.
   - Say it once again.
   - Stick out your tongue.
   - Swallow please.
   - Take a deep breath.
   - Breathe normally.
   - Grasp my hand.
   - Try again.
   - Bear down as if you were to have a bowel movement
     (Valsalva's maneuver).
   - Please lie on your tummy (prone position).
   - Please turn over and lie on your back.
   - Roll over onto your right/left side.
   - Bend your knees.
   - Keep your right knee bent.
   - Lean forward.
   - Get off the couch and stand up.
   - Walk across the room.
   - You can get dressed now. Don't hurry. Take your time.

Table 2. Common phrases used by patients, and their meaning

When a patient says...	The doctor understands...
I can't breath or I'm stuffed up or my chest is tight	Dyspnea
Everything is spinning	Vertigo
It itches me	Pruritus
It stings when I pee	Dysuria
I can't eat or I've lost my appetite	Anorexia
I don't feel like doing anything	Asthenia
Headache	Cephalgia
My nose is dripping	Rhinorrhea
I've vaginal dripping	Leukorrhea
I'm having my period	Menstruation
My hair is falling out	Alopecia
I can't remember a thing	Amnesia
My skin looks yellow	Jaundice
I can't move (a limb)	Paralysis
I can't see anything	Blindness
Bad breath	Halitosis
I've a cavity	Caries
It hurts when I swallow	Odynophagia
I can't swallow	Dysphagia
I spit out phlegm (when I cough)	Sputum
Cough up blood	Hemoptysis
My stomach is burning	Epigastralgia
I wheeze	Wheeze
I've a prickly sensation	Paresthesia
I've a burning sensation	Pyrosis
I feel like I'm going to throw up	Nausea
I'm always running to the bathroom	Polyuria
I always feel like I have to pee	Tenesmus
I'm always thirsty or I'm always dry	Polydipsia
I've a rash	Erythema
My... is swollen	Edema
My skin looks blue	Cyanosis
My chest feels constricted	Thoracic pain
My mouth is always watering	Sialorrhea
I can't breath when I lie down	Orthopnea
My stool is black	Melena
My stool is white	Acholia
My urine is dark	Choluria
I can't sleep	Insomnia
I can't go to the bathroom	Anuria
Bruise	Hematoma
Toothache	Odontalgia

Common Symptom Areas

Pain

- Questions:
  - Which part of your (head, arm, face, chest, ...) is affected?
  - Where does it hurt?
  - Where is it sore?
  - Can you describe the pain?
  - What is the pain like?
  - Is your pain severe?
  - What kind of pain is yours?
  - Is there anything that makes it better?
  - Does anything make it worse?
  - Does anything relieve the pain?
  - What effect does food have?
  - Does lying down help the pain?

- Describing the characteristics of pain:
  - A dull sort of pain.
  - A feeling of pressure.
  - Very sore, like a knife.
  - A burning pain.
  - A gnawing kind of pain.
  - A sharp, stabbing pain.
  - Raw.
  - The pain's gone.
  - A sharp pain.
  - I ache all over.
  - I'm in a lot of pain.
  - I've got a very sore arm.

Fever

- I think I have a temperature.
- I think I'm running a fever.
- High fever.
- High temperature.
- When do you have the highest temperature?
- Do you shiver?
- Were you cold last night?
- When does your temperature come down?

Sickness

- I feel queasy.
- I feel sick.
- I think I'm going to vomit.
- I think I'm going to throw everything up.
- I think I'm going to bring up.
- My head is swimming.
- I feel dizzy.
- He's feeling giddy.
- She's feeling faint.

Weakness

- I feel weak.
- I'm tired.
- I'm not in the mood for ...
- Are you hungry?
- I've lost weight.
- Do you still feel very weak?

Sleep

- Do you feel sleepy?
- Do you sleep deeply?
- I wake up too early.
- Do you snore?

Vision

- I can't see properly.
- Everything is fuzzy.
- I can't see with my left/right eye.
- My eye is itchy.
- My eye is stinging/burning.
- What have you done to your eye?
- What's happened to your eye?

Others

- Have you had a cough?
- Do you pass any blood?
- Do you have a discharge?
- My foot has gone to sleep.
- The patient went into a coma.

Key Words About Symptoms and Signs

General Symptoms

- Malaise
- Anorexia (no appetite)
- Weakness
- Vomiting (throw up)
- Myalgia
- Muscle pain
- Sweats
- Weight loss
- Weight gain
- Drowsiness
- Night sweats
- Insomnia
- Chills
- Numbness
- Tingling
- Fever
- Constipation
- Regular movements
- Diarrhea

Skin

- Rash
- Lump
- Pruritus
- Itch
- Scar
- Bruising
- Spots
- Blackhead
- Moles
- Swelling
- Puffiness
- Tingle

Respiratory System

- Cough
- Productive cough
- Unproductive cough
- Hemoptysis

- Cough up blood
- Cough up phlegm or spit
- Coryza
- Runny nose
- Sputum
- Sore throat
- Pleuritic pain
- Dyspnea
- Breathlessness
- Out of puff
- Chest pain
- Orthopnea
- Breathless on lying down

Cardiovascular System

- Chest pain
- Pain behind the breast bone
- Intermittent claudication
- Cramps
- Palpitations
- Angina
- Tachycardia
- Cyanosis

Gastrointestinal System

- Abdominal pain
- Nausea
- Vomitus
- Vomit
- Diarrhea
- Constipation
- Flatulence
- A coated tongue

Genitourinary System

- Polyuria
- Dysuria
- Pollakiuria
- Tenesmus
- Leukorrhea
- Menorrhagia
- Dysmenorrhea
- Impotence

- Frigidity
- Menstrual cramps

Nervous System

- Tremor
- Rigidity
- Seizure
- Paralysis
- Palsy
- Paresthesia
- Reflex
- Ataxia
- Incontinence
- Jumbled speech
- Knee jerk

Patient Examination

Initial Examination

Level of Consciousness

- Altered level of consciousness
- GCS (Glasgow coma scale)
- Loss of consciousness
- Alert and oriented

Circulation

- Heart tones/sounds
- Clear
- Distant
- Regular/Irregular
- Muffled
- Pulse

Breathing

- Rhythm
- Depth
  - Adequate
  - Shallow
  - Deep

- Quality
  - Easy
  - Labored
  - Stridor
  - Painful
- Shortness of breath

Systematic Examination

Respiratory System

- Breathing
  - Regular
  - Easy
  - Shallow
  - Deep
- Non-productive cough
- Productive cough
- Chest auscultation
- Mucus and pink nail beds
- Telltale stains

Cardiovascular System

- No abnormalities in heart rate or rhythm
- Peripheral pulses
- Normal color and temperature of skin
- No ankle edema

Gastrointestinal System

- Abdomen soft, non-tender
- No nausea or vomiting
- No abnormalities in stool patterns or characteristics
- No change in dietary patterns
- Bowel sounds present

Genitourinary System

- No abnormalities in voiding patterns
- No abnormalities in color or characteristics of urine
- No vaginal or penile drainage

Nervous System

- Finger to finger
- Finger to nose

Special Examinations and Laboratory Findings

Biochemistry

- Prothrombin
- Fibrinogen
- Erythrocyte sedimentation rate (ESR)
- Glucose
- Urea
- Creatinine
- Ion
- Amylase
- Calcium
- Phosphate
- Aspartate aminotransferase (AST)
- Alanine aminotransferase (ALT)
- Alkaline phosphatase
- Urate
- Triglycerides
- Cholesterol
- Creatine kinase (CK)
- LDH (lactate dehydrogenase)
- Iron
- Direct reacting bilirubin (conjugated bilirubin)
- Indirect reacting bilirubin (unconjugated bilirubin)
- Proteins
- Albumin

Hemogram

- Red blood cells
- Hemoglobin
- Hematocrit
- Mean cell volume (MCV)
- Leukocytes
- Neutrophils
- Eosinophils
- Basophils

- Platelets
- Capillary blood sampling

Diagnosis

- Radiography
- Echography/ultrasonography
- Arteriography
- Digitally subtracted angiography (DSA)
- Mammography
- Barium enema
- Double contrast enema
- Urography
- Antegrade urography
- Retrograde urography
- Magnetic resonance (MR)
- Magnetic resonance angiography (MRA)
- Computed tomography (CT)
- Computed tomography angiography (CTA)
- Intravenous urography
- Endoscopy
- Bronchoscopy
- Nuclear medicine
- Spirometry
- Ergometry

Case History

Mr. Wildgoose, a retired bus driver, was unwell and in bed with a cough and *general malaise* when he called in his *general practitioner* (GP). An *upper respiratory tract infection* was diagnosed and erythromycin prescribed. Two days later, on a second home visit, he was found to be a little *breathless* and complaining he felt worse. He was advised to drink plenty and continue with his antibiotic. Another two days passed and the general practitioner returned to find the patient *barely rousable* and *breathless at rest. Emergency admission* to hospital was arranged *on the grounds of* "severe chest infection". *On arrival on the ward*, he was unable to give any history but it was *ascertained* from his wife that he had been confused and unable to get up for the previous 24 hours. He had been incontinent on several occasions during that time. He had been noted to have had increased thirst and nocturia during the previous two weeks.

His past history included appendicectomy at age 12, cervical spondylosis 10 years previously, and hypertension for which he had been taking a thiazide diuretic for three years. His father had died at 62 of myocardial infarction and his mother had had rheumatoid arthritis. His wife *kept* generally *well* but had also had a throat infection the previous week. Mr. Wildgoose drank little alcohol and had stopped smoking two years previously.

Find and underline the phrases providing information on the following:

- Previous occupation
- Initial symptoms
- Initial diagnosis
- Condition prior to admission
- Reason for emergency admission
- Symptoms and their duration from his immediate past history
- Past history
- Family history

Create a new similar case.

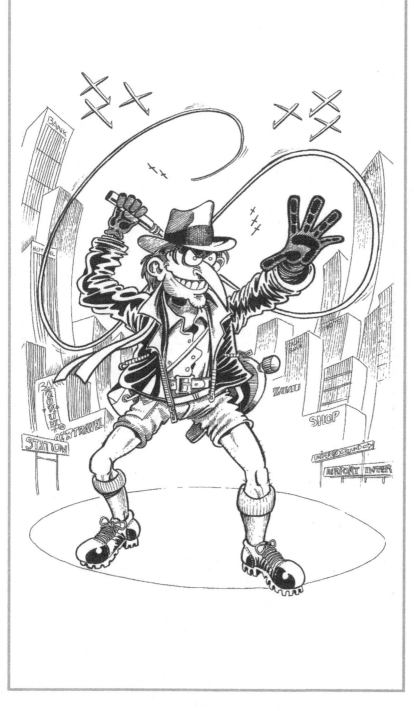

Unit IX Conversation Survival Guide

Introduction

Fluency gives self-confidence and its lack undermines you.

The intention of this chapter is not to replace conversation guides; on the contrary, we encourage you, according to your level, to use them.

Without including translations, it would have been foolish to write a conversation guide. Why, then, have we written this chapter? The aim of the chapter is to provide a "survival guide", a basic tool, to be reviewed by upper-intermediate speakers who actually are perfectly able to understand all the usual exchanges but can have some difficulty in finding natural ways to express themselves in certain unusual scenarios. For instance, we are strolling with a colleague who wants us to accompany him to a jeweler's to buy a bracelet for his wife. Bear in mind that, even in your own language, fluency is virtually impossible in all situations. I have only been upset and disappointed (in English) three times. At a laundry, at an airport, and, on a third occasion, at a restaurant. I considered myself relatively fluent in English by that time but, under pressure, thoughts come to mind much faster than words and your level of fluency can be overwhelmed as a consequence of the adrenaline levels of your blood. Accept this piece of advice: unless you are bilingual you cannot afford to get into arguments in a language other than your own.

Many upper-intermediate speakers do not take a conversation guide when traveling abroad. They think their level is well above those who need a guide to construct basic sentences and are ashamed of being seen reading one (I myself went through this stage). I was (and they are) utterly wrong in not taking a guide because, for upper-intermediate speakers, a conversation guide has different and very important uses (as my level increased, I realized that my use of these guides changed; I did not need to read the translations, except for a few words, and I just looked for natural ways of saying things).

In my opinion, even being bilingual, conversation guides are extremely helpful whenever you are in an unfamiliar environment such as, for example, a florist. How many names of flowers do you know in your own language? Probably less than a dozen. Think that every conversation scenario has its own jargon and a conversation guide can give you the hints that an upper-intermediate speaker may need to be actually fluent in many situations. So, do not be ashamed of carrying and reading a guide, even in public; they are the shortest way to fluency in those unfamiliar scenarios that sporadically test our English level and, what is more important, our self-confidence in English.

Whenever you have to go out to dinner, for example, review the key words and usual sentences of your conversation guide. It will not take more than ten minutes, and your dinner will taste even better since you have ordered it with unbelievable fluency and precision. What is just a recommendable task for upper-intermediate speakers is absolutely mandatory for lower-intermediate speakers who, before leaving the hotel, should review, and rehearse the sentences they will need to ask for whatever they want to eat or, at least, to avoid ordering what they never would eat in their own country. Looking at the faces of your colleagues once the first course is served you will realize who is eating what he wanted and who, on the contrary, does not know what he ordered and, what is worse, what he is actually eating.

Let us think for a moment about this incident that happened to me when I was at UCSF Medical Center. I was invited to have lunch at a diner near the hospital, and when I asked for still mineral water, the somewhat surprised waiter answered that they did not have still mineral water but sparkling because no customer had ever asked for such a "delicacy" and offered me plain water instead. (If you do not understand this story, the important words to look up in the dictionary are *diner* (with one "n"), *still*, *sparkling* and *plain*.)

Would you be fluent without the help of a guide in a car breakdown? I did have a leak in the gas tank on a trip with my wife and mother-in-law from Boston to Niagara Falls and Toronto. I still remember the face of the mechanic in Toronto when asking me if we were staying in downtown Toronto. I answered that we were on our way back to ... Boston. I can tell you that my worn guide was vital, without it I would not have been able to explain what the problem was. This was the last time I had to take the guide from a hidden pocket in my suitcase. Since then I have kept my guide with me, even at ... the beach, because unexpected situations may arise at any time by definition. Think of possibly embarrassing, although not infrequent, situations and ... do not forget your guide on your next trip abroad (the inside pocket of your jacket is a suitable place for those who still have not overcome the stage of "guide-ashamedness").

Those who have reached a certain level are aware of the many embarrassing situations they have had to overcome in the past to become fluent in a majority of circumstances.

At the Airport

Here are some common sentences to review:

- I'll wait for you in the departure lounge.
- Our flight to Madrid has been cancelled because of the snow.
- How soon should we be at the airport before take-off?
- How can I get to the airport?
- What weight am I allowed?
- What time does the plane to Chicago leave?
- Passengers for flight number 112 to Amsterdam go to gate 7.
- Hurry up! We have been called over the loudspeaker.
- Pick up your luggage at the terminal.
- One of my suitcases has been lost.
- Flight number 112 to Paris has been cancelled.
- Do you have anything to declare? No I don't.
- Do you have anything to declare? Yes, I am a doctor and I'm carrying some surgical instruments.
- Do you have anything to declare? Yes, I have bought six bottles of whisky and four cartons of cigarettes in the duty free.
- I have misplaced my hand luggage. Where is lost property?
- How much more would I need to pay if I wanted to upgrade this ticket to first class?
- I want to change the return flight date from Boston to Madrid to November 30th.
- My luggage is overweight. How much more do I need to pay?
- I want to buy a flight ticket to London leaving this afternoon. Is there a direct flight or not? Is it via Zurich?
- Is it possible to purchase an open ticket?
- I have missed my flight to New York. Would you please tell me when the next flight leaves? Can I use the ticket I have or do I need to pay for a new one?

During the Flight

Very few exchanges are likely during a normal flight. Being familiar with them you will feel how fluency interferes positively with your mood. Conversely, if you need a pillow and are not able to ask for it, your self-confidence will shrink, your neck will hurt, and you will not ask for anything else during the flight. On my first flight to the States I did not know how to ask for a pillow and tried to convince myself that I did not actually need one. When I looked it up in my guide, asked for it, and the stewardess brought the pillow, I gladly and pleasantly fell asleep.

Do not let lack of fluency spoil an otherwise perfect flight.

- Is there an aisle seat free? (I asked for one at the check-in and they told me I should ask on board just in case there had been a cancellation.)
- Is there a window seat free?
- Would you please bring me a blanket/pillow?
- Can I visit the cockpit? The captain is a friend of mine.
- Is there a business class seat free?
- Can I upgrade my ticket to first class on board?
- Is there a vegetarian menu?
- Stewardess, I'm feeling bad. Do you have anything for flight-sickness?
- Stewardess, this gentleman is disturbing me.

In the Taxi

Think for a moment of taking a taxi in your city. How many sentences are supposed to be exchanged in normal, and even extraordinary, conditions? I assure you that with fewer than two dozen sentences you will solve more than ninety per cent of possible situations.

- Where is the nearest taxi rank?
- Would you call a taxi for me? (At the hotel)
- Hi, take me to the Metropolitan, please.
- Would you please take me to Trafalgar Square?
- Which way do you want me to take you, via Fifth or Seventh Avenue? Either one would be OK.
- I'm in a hurry!
- Would you mind putting your cigarette out?
- Stop at number 112, please.
- Pull over, I'll be back in a minute.
- Is there any surcharge to the airport?
- Stop here.
- Would you mind not smoking please?
- Would you please wind your window up? I am a little bit cold.
- Is the air conditioning on?
- How much is it?
- How much do I owe you?
- Is the tip included?
- Would you give me a receipt?
- This is too expensive.
- They have never charged me this before. Give me a receipt; I'll make a complaint.

At the Hotel

Checking In

Here are some sentences that may be useful during check in:

- Hello, I have reserved a room under the name of Dr. Viamonte.
- Do you need my ID?
- Do you need my credit card?
- Can you double-check that we have a double room with a view of the beach?
- I want a double bed.
- I want a single bed.
- I asked for two single beds.
- Is breakfast included?
- Is there anybody who can help me with my bags?
- Could you recommend a good restaurant near to the hotel?
- Does the hotel have a car park?
- Do you have a car park nearby?

The Stay

Here are some sentences that may be useful during your stay:

- Can you give me a wake-up call at seven each morning?
- There is no hot water. Would you please send someone to fix it?
- The TV is not working properly. Would you please send some one to fix it?
- The bathtub has no plug. Would you please send someone up with one.
- The people in the room next to mine are making a racket. Would you please tell them to keep it down?
- I want to change my room. It is too noisy.
- I need an extra bed.
- What time does breakfast start?
- How can I get to the city center?
- Can we change dollars?
- Could you recommend a good restaurant?
- Would you give me the room service number?
- I will have a cheese omelet, a ham sandwich, and an orange juice.

Checking Out

Here are some sentences that may be useful when checking out:

- How much is it?
- Can I pay in dollars?
- Would you please call a taxi?
- Do you accept credit cards?
- There is a mistake in the receipt:
  - I have had only one breakfast.
  - I thought breakfast was included.
  - I have been in a single room.
- Can you give me the complaints book?
- Would you please give me the keys to my car?
- Is there anybody here who can help me with my luggage?

At the Restaurant

"The same for me" is one of the most common sentences heard at tables around the world. The non-fluent English speaker links his/her gastronomic fate to a reportedly more fluent one in order to avoid uncomfortable counter-questions such as "How would you like your meat, sir?"

A simple look at a guide a few minutes before the dinner will provide you with enough vocabulary to ask for whatever you want.

Do not let your lack of fluency spoil a good opportunity to taste delicious dishes or wines.

Preliminary Exchanges

- Hello, have you got a table for three people?
- Hi, may I book a table for a party of seven at 6 o'clock?
- What time are you coming, sir?
- Where can we sit?
- Is this chair free?
- Is this table taken?
- Waiter/waitress I would like to order.
- Could I see the menu?
- Could you bring the menu?
- Can I have the wine list?
- Could you give us a table next to the window?
- Could you give me a table on the mezzanine?
- Could you give us a table near the stage?

Ordering

- We'd like to order now.
- Could you bring us some bread, please?
- The same for me.
- We'd like to have something to drink.
- Here you are.
- Enjoy your meal, sir.
- Could you recommend a local wine?
- Could you recommend one of your specialties?
- Could you suggest something special?
- What are the ingredients of this dish?
- I'll have a steamed lobster, please.
- Excuse me, I have spilt something on my tie. Could you help me?
- How would you like your meat, sir?
- Rare/medium-rare/medium/well-done.
- Is the halibut fresh?
- Somewhere between rare and medium rare will be OK.
- What is there for dessert?
- Anything else, sir?
- No, we are fine, thank you.
- How was everything, sir?
- The meal was excellent.
- The sirloin was delicious.

Complaining

- The dish is cold. Would you please heat it up?
- The meat is underdone. Would you cook it a little more, please?
- Excuse me. This is not what I asked for.
- Could you change this for me?
- The fish is not fresh. I want to see the manager.
- I asked for a sirloin.
- The meal wasn't very good.
- The meat smells off.
- Could you bring the complaints book?
- This wine is off, I think ...
- Waiter, this fork is dirty.

The Check (the Bill)

- The check, please.
- Would you bring us the check, please?
- All together, please.
- We are paying separately.
- I am afraid there is a mistake, we didn't have this.
- This is for you.
- Keep the change.

Shopping

Preliminary Exchanges

- Hello sir (madam), may I help you?
- Hi, do you sell ...?
- I am looking for a ... Can you help me?
- Would you tell me where the record department is?
- On which floor is the leather goods department?
- On the ground floor (on the mezzanine, on the second floor ...)
- Would you please show me ...?
- What kind do you want?

Buying Clothes/Shoes

- Please, can you show me some natural silk ties?
- I want to buy a long-sleeved shirt.
- I want the pair of high-heeled shoes I have seen in the window.
- Would you please show me the pair in the window?
- What material is it?
- What material is it made of?
  - Cotton
  - Leather
  - Linen
  - Wool
  - Velvet
  - Silk
  - Nylon
  - Acrylic fiber
- What size, please?
- Is this my size?
- Do you think this is my size?
- Where is the fitting room?

- Does it fit you?
- I think it fits well although the collar is a little tight.
- No, it doesn't fit me.
- May I try a larger size?
- I'll try a smaller size. Would you bring it to me?
- I'll take this one.
- How much is it?
- This is too expensive.
- Oh, this is a bargain!
- I like it.
- May I try this on?
- In which color?
- Navy blue, please.

At the Bookshop

- I would like to buy a book on the history of the city.
- Is the book translated into Japanese?
- Have you got Swedish newspapers/magazines?
- Where can I buy a road map?

Developing Photos

- I want a 36 exposure film for this camera.
- Could you develop this film?
- How much does developing cost?
- When will the photographs be ready?
- My camera is not working, would you have a look at it?
- Do you take passport (ID) photographs?
- I want an enlargement of this one and two copies of this other.

At the Florist

- I would like to order a bouquet of roses.
- You can choose violets and orchids in several colors.
- What are these flowers called?
- Could you please send this bouquet to the NH Abascal hotel manager at 47 Abascal St. before noon?

Paying

- Where is the cash machine?
- How much is that all together?
- Will you pay cash or by credit card?
- Next in line (queue).
- Could you gift-wrap it for me?

At the Hairdresser

When I was in Boston I went to a hairdresser's and my lack of fluency was responsible for a drastic change in my image for a couple of months so that my wife almost did not recognize me when I picked her up at Logan on one of her multiple visits to New England. I can assure you that I will never forget the word "sideburns"; the hairdresser, a robust Afro-American lady, drastically cut them before I could recall the name of this insignificant part of my facial hair. To tell you the truth, I did not know how important sideburns were until I didn't have them.

If you do not trust an unknown hairdresser, "just a trim" would be a polite way of avoiding a disaster.

I recommend, before going to the hairdresser, a thorough review of your guide so that you get familiar with key words such as: *scissors, comb, brush, dryer, shampooing, hair style, manicure, dyeing, beard, moustache, sideboards*(!), *fringe, curl* or *plait*.

Men and Women

- How long will I have to wait?
- Is the water OK?
- It is fine/too hot/too cold.
- My hair is greasy/dry.
- I have dandruff.
- A shampoo, please.
- How would you like it?
- I want a (hair)cut like this.
- However you want.
- Is it OK?
- That's fine, thank you.

Men

- A razor cut, please.
- I want a shave.
- Just a trim.
- Leave the sideburns as they are(!) – (UK sideboards)
- Trim the moustache.
- Towards the back, without any parting.

Women

- How do I set your hair?
- What hair style do you want?
- I would like to dye my hair.
- Same color?
- A little darker/lighter.
- I would like to have a perm (permanent wave).

Cars

As always, begin with key words. *Clutch, brake, blinkers, trunk* (UK *boot*), *tank, gearbox, windshield* (UK *windscreen*) *wipers, (steering) wheel, unleaded gas* (UK *petrol*), etc, must belong to your fund of knowledge of English as well as several usual sentences such as:

- How far is the nearest gas (petrol) station?
- In what direction?

At the Petrol Station

- Fill it up, please.
- Unleaded, please.
- Could you top up the battery, please?
- Could you check the oil, please?
- Could you check the tyre pressures, please?
- Do you want me to check the spare tyre too?

At the Garage

- My car has broken down.
- What's wrong with the car?
- Could you mend this puncture?
- Can you take the car in tow to downtown Boston?
- I see ..., kill the engine, please.
- Start the engine, please.
- The car goes to the right and overheats.
- Have you noticed if it loses water/gas/oil?
- Yes, it's loosing oil.
- Does it lose speed?
- Yes, and it doesn't start properly.
- I can't get it into reverse.
- The motor makes funny noises.
- Please, repair it as soon as possible.
- I wonder if you can fix it temporarily.
- How long will it take to repair it?
- I am afraid we have to send for spare parts.
- The car drinks too much.
- I want to change the right front tyre.
- I guess the valve is broken.
- Have you finished fixing the car?
- Did you fix the car?

At the Car Park

- Is there a car park near here?
- Are there any free spaces?
- How much is it per hour?
- Is the car park supervised?
- How long can I leave the car here?

Renting a Car

- I want to rent a car.
- For how many days?
- Unlimited mileage?
- What is the cost per mile?
- Is insurance included?
- You should leave a deposit.

How Can I Get To ...?

- How far is Minneapolis?
- It is not far. About 12 miles from here.
- Is the road good?
- It is not bad, although a bit slow.
- There are many bends.
- Is there a toll road between here and Berlin?
- How long does it take to get to Key West?
- I am lost. Could you tell me how I can get back to the toll road.

Having a Drink (or Two)

Nothing is more desirable than a drink after a hard day of meetings. In such a relaxed situation embarrassing incidents can happen. Often, there is a difficult counter-question to a simple "Can I have a beer?" such as "would you prefer lager?" or "small, medium or large, sir?". From my own experience, when I was a beginner, I hated counter-questions and I remember my face flushing when in a pub in London, instead of giving me the beer I asked for, the barman responded with the entire list of beers in the pub. "I have changed my mind, I'll have a Coke instead" was my response to both "the aggression" I suffered from the barman and the embarrassment resulting from my lack of fluency. "We don't serve Coke here, sir." These situations can spoil the most promising evening so ... let's review a bunch of usual sentences:
- Two beers please, my friend will pay.
- Where is there a good place to go for a drink?
- Where can we go for a drink at this time of the evening?
- Do you know any pubs with live music?
- What can I get you?
- A glass of wine and two beers, please.
- A gin and tonic.
- A glass of brandy. Would you please warm the glass?
- Scotch, please.
- Do you want it plain, with water, or on the rocks?
- Make it a double.
- I'll have the same again, please.
- Two cubes of ice please and a teaspoon.
- This is on me.
- What those ladies are having is on me.

On the Phone

Many problems start when you lift the receiver. You hear a continuous purring different from the one you are used to in your country or a strange sequence of rapid pips. Immediately "what the hell am I supposed to do right now" comes to your mind, and we face one of the most embarrassing situations for non-fluent speakers. The phone has two added difficulties: firstly, its immediacy and, secondly, the absence of image ("if I could see this guy I would understand what he was saying"). Do not worry, the preliminary exchanges in this conversational scenario are few. Answering machines are another different, and tougher, problem and are out of the scope of this survival guide. Just a tip: do not hang up. Try to catch what the machine is saying and give it another try in case you are not able to follow its instructions. Many doctors, as soon as they hear the unmistakable sound of these devices, terrified, hang up thinking they are too much for them. Most messages are much easier to understand and less mechanical than those given by "human" (and usually bored) operators.

- Where are the public phones, please?
- Where is the nearest call-box?
- Operator, what do I dial for the USA?
- Hold on a moment … number one.
- Would you get me this number please?
- Dial straight through.
- What time does the cheap rate begin?
- Have you got any phone cards, please?
- Can I use your cell phone, please?
- Do you have a phone book (directory)?
- I'd like to make a reverse charge call to Korea.
- The line is engaged.
- There's no answer.
- It's a bad line.
- I've been cut off.

In the Bank

Nowadays, the spread of credit cards makes this section virtually unnecessary but, in my experience, when things go really bad you may need to go to a bank. Fluency disappears in stressful situations so, in case you have to solve a bank problem, review not only this bunch of sentences but the entire section in your guide.

- Where can I change money?
- I'd like to change 200 Euros.

- I want to change 1000 Euros into Dollars/Pounds.
- Could I have it in tens, please?
- What's the exchange rate?
- What's the rate of exchange from Euros to Dollars?
- What are the banking hours?
- I want to change this traveler's check.
- Have you received a transfer from Rosario Nadal addressed to Fiona Shaw?
- Can I cash this bearer check?
- I want to cash this check.
- Do I need my ID to cash this bearer check?
- Go to the cash desk.
- Go to counter number 5.
- May I open a current account?
- Where is the nearest cash machine?
- I am afraid you are not able to solve my problem, can I see the manager?
- Who is in charge?
- Could you call my bank in France? There must have been a problem with a transfer addressed to myself.